Diverticulitis

Table of Content

Chapter 1: Understanding Diverticulitis Disease 1
- What is Diverticulitis? 1
- Relation Between Diverticulitis and Diverticulitis 1
- The Causes 1
- Signs and Symptoms 2
- Risk Factors 2
- Diagnosis 2

Chapter 2: Diverticulitis Complications 4
- Abscess 4
- Perforation 4
- Peritonitis 4
- Rectal Bleeding 5
- Fistula 5
- Intestinal Obstruction 5

Chapter 3: Diverticulitis Treatment Options 6
- Diet 6
- The Healing Diverticulitis Diet 6
- Antibiotics 10
- CT Scan-Guided Percutaneous Drainage 10
- Surgery 11
- Risks of Surgery 12
- What to Expect After the Surgery 12
- After Discharge Expectations and Guidelines 12

Chapter 4: Diet Guide for Diverticulitis 13
- Stage 1: The Clear Liquid Diet 13
- Stage 2: The Juicing Diet 15
- Stage 3: The Low Residue Diet 16
- Stage 4: The High Fiber Diet 17

THE 4 PHASE DIET RECIPES 19

Chapter 1: Understanding Diverticulitis Disease

What is Diverticulitis?

Diverticulitis is a common digestive disease which involves the formation of pouches (diverticula) within the bowel wall. This process is known as diverticulosis, and typically occurs within the large intestine, or colon, although it can occasionally occur in the small intestine as well. Diverticulitis results when one of these diverticula becomes inflamed.

People often have pain in the left lower area of the intestine, abdominal pain and tenderness, fever and an increased white blood cell count. They may also complain of nausea or diarrhea; others may be constipated. The severity of symptoms depends on the extent of the infection and complications. Less commonly, an individual with diverticulitis may have right-sided abdominal pain. This may be due to the less common right-sided diverticula or a highly redundant sigmoid colon. Some patients report bleeding from the rectum.

Relation Between Diverticulitis and Diverticulitis

This process of the formation of pouches within the bowel wall is known as diverticulitis, and typically occurs within the large intestine, or colon, although it can occasionally occur in the small intestine as well. Diverticulitis results when one of these diverticulitis becomes inflamed.

The Causes

The causes of diverticulitis are poorly understood, with approximately 40% due to genetics and 60% due to environmental factors. Obesity is another risk factor.

Signs and Symptoms
People often have pain in the left lower area of the intestine, abdominal pain and tenderness, fever and an increased white blood cell count. They may also complain of nausea or diarrhea; others may be constipated. The severity of symptoms depends on the extent of the infection and complications. Less commonly, an individual with diverticulitis may have right-sided abdominal pain. This may be due to the less common right-sided diverticula or a highly redundant sigmoid colon. Some patients report bleeding from the rectum.

Risk Factors
The risk factors are obesity, genetics, environmental.

Diagnosis
People with the above symptoms are commonly studied with computed tomography, or CT scan. The CT scan is very accurate (98%) in diagnosing diverticulitis. In order to extract the most information possible about the patient's condition, thin section (5 mm) transverse images are obtained through the entire abdomen and pelvis after the patient has been administered oral and intravascular contrast. Images reveal localized colon wall thickening, with inflammation extending into the fat surrounding the colon. The diagnosis of acute diverticulitis is made confidently when the involved segment contains diverticula. CT may also identify patients with more complicated diverticulitis, such as those with an associated abscess. It may even allow for radiologically guided drainage of an associated abscess, sparing a patient from immediate surgical intervention.

To diagnose diverticular disease, the doctor asks about medical history, does a physical exam, and may perform one or more diagnostic tests. Because most people do not have symptoms, diverticulosis is often found through tests ordered for another ailment. For example, diverticulosis is often found during a colonoscopy done to screen for cancer or polyps or to evaluate complaints of pain or rectal bleeding.

When taking a medical history, the doctor may ask about bowel habits, pain, other symptoms, diet, and medications. The physical exam usually involves a digital rectal exam. To perform this test, the doctor inserts a gloved, lubricated finger into the rectum to detect tenderness, blockage, or blood. The doctor may check stool for signs of bleeding and test blood for signs of infection. If diverticulitis is suspected, the doctor may order one of the following radiologic tests:

- **Abdominal ultrasound.** Sound waves are sent toward the colon through a handheld device that a technician glides over the abdomen. The sound waves bounce off the colon and other organs, and their echoes make electrical impulses that create a picture-called a sonogram-on a video monitor. If the diverticula are inflamed, the sound waves will also bounce off of them, showing their location.

- **Computerized tomography (CT) scan.** The CT scan is a noninvasive x ray that produces cross-section images of the body. The doctor may inject dye into a vein and the person may be given a similar mixture to swallow. The person lies on a table that slides into a donut-shaped machine. The dye helps to show complications of diverticulitis such as perforations and abscesses.

Other studies, such as barium enema and colonoscopy are contraindicated in the acute phase of diverticulitis because of the risk of perforation.

Most cases of simple, uncomplicated diverticulitis respond to conservative therapy with bowel rest.

Chapter 2: Diverticulitis Complications

Abscess

Diverticulitis may lead to infection, which often clears up after a few days of treatment with antibiotics. If the infection gets worse, an abscess may form in the wall of the colon.

An abscess is a localized collection of pus that may cause swelling and destroy tissue. If the abscess is small and remains in the wall of the colon, it may clear up after treatment with antibiotics. If the abscess does not clear up with antibiotics, the doctor may need to drain it using a catheter-a small tube-placed into the abscess through the skin. After giving the patient numbing medicine, the doctor inserts the needle through the skin until reaching the abscess and then drains the fluid through the catheter. This process may be guided by sonography or x ray.

Perforation

Infected diverticula may develop perforations. Sometimes the perforations leak pus out of the colon and form a large abscess in the abdominal cavity, a condition called peritonitis. A person with peritonitis may be extremely ill with nausea, vomiting, fever, and severe abdominal tenderness. The condition requires immediate surgery to clean the abdominal cavity and remove the damaged part of the colon. Without prompt treatment, peritonitis can be fatal.

Peritonitis

Infected diverticula may develop perforations. Sometimes the perforations leak pus out of the colon and form a large abscess in the abdominal cavity, a condition called peritonitis. A person with peritonitis may be extremely ill with nausea, vomiting, fever, and severe abdominal tenderness. The condition requires immediate surgery to clean the abdominal cavity and remove the damaged part of the colon. Without prompt treatment, peritonitis can be fatal.

Rectal Bleeding

Rectal bleeding from diverticula is a rare complication. Doctors believe the bleeding is caused by a small blood vessel in a diverticulum that weakens and then bursts. When diverticula bleed, blood may appear in the toilet or in the stool. Bleeding can be severe, but it may stop by itself and not require treatment. A person who has bleeding from the rectum-even a small amount-should see a doctor right away. Often, colonoscopy is used to identify the site of bleeding and stop the bleeding. Sometimes the doctor injects dye into an artery-a procedure called angiography-to identify and treat diverticular bleeding. If the bleeding does not stop, surgery may be necessary to remove the involved portion of the colon.

Fistula

A fistula is an abnormal connection of tissue between two organs or between an organ and the skin. When damaged tissues come into contact with each other during infection, they sometimes stick together. If they heal that way, a fistula may form. When diverticulitis-related infection spreads outside the colon, the colon's tissue may stick to nearby tissues. The organs usually involved are the bladder, small intestine, and skin.

The most common type of fistula occurs between the bladder and the colon. This type of fistula affects men more often than women. It can result in a severe, long-lasting infection of the urinary tract. The problem can be corrected with surgery to remove the fistula and the affected part of the colon.

Intestinal Obstruction

Scarring caused by infection may lead to partial or total blockage of the intestine, called intestinal obstruction. When the intestine is blocked, the colon is unable to move bowel contents normally. If the intestine is completely blocked, emergency surgery is necessary. Partial blockage is not an emergency, so the surgery to correct it can be planned.

Chapter 3: Diverticulitis Treatment Options

Diet

People may be placed on a low residue diet. It was previously thought that a low-fiber diet gives the colon adequate time to heal. Evidence tends to run counter to this with a 2011 review finding no evidence for the superiority of low residue diets in treating diverticular disease and that a high-fiber diet may prevent diverticular disease. A systematic review published in 2012 found no high quality studies, but found that some studies and guidelines favor a high-fiber diet for the treatment of symptomatic disease.

The Healing Diverticulitis Diet

During a diverticulitis flare-up, or at first symptoms, it is important to help your digestive tract clean itself out, and begin to heal. Start by using my beef bone broth recipe.

Eating bone broths made from beef, chicken, lamb and fish helps to heal leaky gut syndrome, improves joint health, boosts the immune system, and even helps to reduce cellulite, all while helping to heal the digestive tract.

Bone broths with cooked vegetables and a little bit of meat, provides essential nutrients your body needs, including calcium, magnesium, phosphorus, silicon, sulphur, and more, in an easily digested manner.

You may add vegetables to your bone broth including carrots, celery and garlic or for variation, you may add an egg poached in the broth. In addition, sip on warm ginger tea two to three times daily to help reduce inflammation and aid in digestion. Ginger is a healing food that helps your immune and digestive systems.

For beef, the collagen in the bones breaks down into gelatin within about 48 hours, and for chicken it is about 24. You can make broth in less time, but to get the most out of the bones, I recommend making it in a crock pot closer to 48 hours.

Gelatin has amazing curative properties and even helps individuals with food sensitivities and allergies tolerate these foods more easily. It also promotes probiotic balance, while breaking down proteins making them easier to digest. The real truth about probiotics is that they help to create a healthy environment in your stomach.

During this first phase of the diverticulitis diet, consume only clear bone broths, clear fresh juices (no pulp), and soothing ginger tea.

When your body has adapted to these foods, start to add fiber rich foods including raw fruits and vegetables, and unrefined grains, such as quinoa, black rice, fermented grains, or sprouted lentils. *It is important to stay away from whole nuts and seeds, as they can easily become trapped in the diverticula, causing further damage.*

According to researchers at the University of Oxford, fiber reduces the risk of diverticular disease. The study focused on fiber from fruits, vegetables, cereals, and potatoes.

So over the first few days, introduce high-fiber foods gradually, adding just one new food every 3-4 days.

As your body starts to adapt you can begin consuming about 25-35 grams of fiber each day, to help stave off any potential flare-ups, while your digestive tract heals. Add in some potatoes, sweet potatoes, root vegetables, then slowly try some non-processed grains or beans such as oats or lentils.

One important distinction is the difference between soluble fiber, and insoluble fiber. Soluble fiber actually retains water, and turns into a gel during the digestive process. The gel helps to slow the digestion, allowing for greater absorption of essential nutrients. Insoluble fiber, on the other hand, adds bulk to stools, allowing foods to more quickly leave your system.

Foods high in soluble fiber include oat bran, nuts, seeds, beans, lentils barley, and peas. Insoluble fiber is found in foods including whole grains, wheat bran, and vegetables.

Researchers at the Department of Nutrition at Harvard Medical School found that it is the insoluble fiber that decreases risk for developing diverticular disease. But do not let this sway you from eating a balanced diet. You do not have to eliminate soluble fiber, nor should you.

Maintaining a healthy balance of protein, fiber, and fresh fruits and vegetables, is essential for keeping diverticulitis from flaring up.

Native Americans have used slippery elm for centuries both externally, and internally to soothe digestive problems and relieve coughs and sore throats.

Today, it is recommended to relieve the symptoms of GERD, Crohn's disease, IBS, and digestive upset. Start by taking 500 milligrams, 3 times daily, throughout the course of the diverticulitis diet. Be sure to take with a full glass of water, or other clear liquid.

Aloe, in a juice form, aids in digestion, helps to normalize pH levels, regularizes bowel processing, and encourages healthy digestive bacteria. It is important to avoid aloe vera juice with "aloe latex", as it can cause severe stomach cramping and diarrhea.

12 to 16 ounces per day of aloe juice is recommended; any more than that can further irritate your system.

You can find it in the organics section of a local grocery store or in many Asian markets.

Licorice Root lowers stomach acid levels, can relieve heartburn, and acts as a mild laxative to help clear your colon of waste. This root helps to increase bile, aiding in digestion, while lowering cholesterol levels. Take 100 milligrams daily when experiencing diverticulitis symptoms.

In addition to healing your colon from diverticulitis, the overall goal of the diverticulitis diet, supplements, and lifestyle changes, is to encourage your digestive tract to function optimally.

Digestive enzymes help break down foods, making it possible to absorb nutrients. Individuals with digestion problems can take digestive supplements that contain essential enzymes to facilitate digestion.

Live probiotics should be added to the diet to help negate food sensitivities, and relieve digestive upset including constipation, gas, and bloating. Probiotics are healthy bacteria that traditionally line your digestive tract to combat infection. If you have diverticulitis you need an influx of these bacteria to aid in the healing of your colon, while preventing disease recurrence.

Diverticulitis requires more than just a healing diverticulitis diet, and supplements to aid in a healthy digestive tract. Digestion starts in the mouth. It is essential to thoroughly chew each bite of food, until it is nearly liquefied. The more you break down the food before it hits the stomach, the more ready nutrients are ready to be absorbed.

Medical studies show that the combination of physical activity and high fiber diets helps to prevent diverticular disease. Running, or using a rebounder daily, helps to relieve symptoms and reduce flare-ups. Even moderate intensity exercise helps to regulate bowel functions, reduces stress, and supports healthy weight.

Your psychological health is an integral part of your wellness; managing stress and learning effective coping mechanisms is essential. Stress affects not only the mind, but the body as well.

Straining while on the toilet creates too much pressure in the colon resulting in small tears. Choose to elevate feet slightly on a stool as this helps to reduce straining.

Antibiotics

Diverticulitis may lead to infection, which often clears up after a few days of treatment with antibiotics. If the infection gets worse, an abscess may form in the wall of the colon.

An abscess is a localized collection of pus that may cause swelling and destroy tissue. If the abscess is small and remains in the wall of the colon, it may clear up after treatment with antibiotics. If the abscess does not clear up with antibiotics, the doctor may need to drain it using a catheter-a small tube-placed into the abscess through the skin. After giving the patient numbing medicine, the doctor inserts the needle through the skin until reaching the abscess and then drains the fluid through the catheter. This process may be guided by sonography or x ray.

CT Scan-Guided Percutaneous Drainage

People with the above symptoms are commonly studied with computed tomography, or CT scan. The CT scan is very accurate (98%) in diagnosing diverticulitis. In order to extract the most information possible about the patient's condition, thin section (5 mm) transverse images are obtained through the entire abdomen and pelvis after the patient has been administered oral and intravascular contrast. Images reveal localized colon wall thickening, with inflammation extending into the fat surrounding the colon. The diagnosis of acute diverticulitis is made confidently when the involved segment contains diverticula. CT may also identify patients with more complicated diverticulitis, such as those with an associated abscess. It may even allow for radiologically guided drainage of an associated abscess, sparing a patient from immediate surgical intervention.

To diagnose diverticular disease, the doctor asks about medical history, does a physical exam, and may perform one or more diagnostic tests. Because most people do not have symptoms, diverticulosis is often found through tests ordered for another ailment. For example, diverticulosis is often found during a colonoscopy done to screen for cancer or polyps or to evaluate complaints of pain or rectal bleeding.

When taking a medical history, the doctor may ask about bowel habits, pain, other symptoms, diet, and medications. The physical exam usually involves a digital rectal exam. To perform this test, the doctor inserts a gloved, lubricated finger into the rectum to detect tenderness, blockage, or blood. The doctor may check stool for signs of bleeding and test blood for signs of infection. If diverticulitis is suspected, the doctor may order the following radiologic test:

Computerized tomography (CT) scan. The CT scan is a noninvasive x ray that produces cross-section images of the body. The doctor may inject dye into a vein and the person may be given a similar mixture to swallow. The person lies on a table that slides into a donut-shaped machine. The dye helps to show complications of diverticulitis such as perforations and abscesses.

Surgery

Severe cases of diverticulitis with acute pain and complications will likely require a hospital stay. When a person has complications or does not respond to medication, surgery may be necessary.

Infected diverticula may develop perforations. Sometimes the perforations leak pus out of the colon and form a large abscess in the abdominal cavity, a condition called peritonitis. A person with peritonitis may be extremely ill with nausea, vomiting, fever, and severe abdominal tenderness. The condition requires immediate surgery to clean the abdominal cavity and remove the damaged part of the colon. Without prompt treatment, peritonitis can be fatal.

Rectal bleeding from diverticula is a rare complication. Doctors believe the bleeding is caused by a small blood vessel in a diverticulum that weakens and then bursts. When diverticula bleed, blood may appear in the toilet or in the stool. Bleeding can be severe, but it may stop by itself and not require treatment. A person who has bleeding from the rectum-even a small amount-should see a doctor right away. Often, colonoscopy is used to identify the site of bleeding and stop the bleeding. Sometimes the doctor injects dye into an artery-a procedure called angiography-to identify and treat diverticular bleeding. If the bleeding does not stop, surgery may be necessary to remove the involved portion of the colon.

The most common type of fistula occurs between the bladder and the colon. This type of fistula affects men more often than women. It can result in a severe, long-lasting infection of the urinary tract. The problem can be corrected with surgery to remove the fistula and the affected part of the colon.

Scarring caused by infection may lead to partial or total blockage of the intestine, called intestinal obstruction. When the intestine is blocked, the colon is unable to move bowel contents normally. If the intestine is completely blocked, emergency surgery is necessary. Partial blockage is not an emergency, so the surgery to correct it can be planned.

Risks of Surgery
As with all surgery, there are affiliated risks and potential complications. You should discuss all risks with your doctor.

What to Expect After the Surgery
As with all surgery, there are affiliated risks and potential complications. You should discuss all risks and healing with your doctor.

After Discharge Expectations and Guidelines
As with all surgery, there are affiliated risks and potential complications. You should discuss all risks and healing with your doctor.

Chapter 4: Diet Guide for Diverticulitis

Stage 1: The Clear Liquid Diet

People may be placed on a low residue diet. It was previously thought that a low-fiber diet gives the colon adequate time to heal. Evidence tends to run counter to this with a 2011 review finding no evidence for the superiority of low residue diets in treating diverticular disease and that a high-fiber diet may prevent diverticular disease. A systematic review published in 2012 found no high quality studies, but found that some studies and guidelines favor a high-fiber diet for the treatment of symptomatic disease.

Goals

During a diverticulitis flare-up, or at first symptoms, it is important to help your digestive tract clean itself out, and begin to heal. Start by using my beef bone broth recipe.

Guidelines for the Clear Liquid Diet

Eating bone broths made from beef, chicken, lamb and fish helps to heal leaky gut syndrome, improves joint health, boosts the immune system, and even helps to reduce cellulite, all while helping to heal the digestive tract.

Bone broths with cooked vegetables and a little bit of meat, provides essential nutrients your body needs, including calcium, magnesium, phosphorus, silicon, sulphur, and more, in an easily digested manner.

You may add vegetables to your bone broth including carrots, celery and garlic or for variation, you may add an egg poached in the broth. In addition, sip on warm ginger tea two to three times daily to help reduce inflammation and aid in digestion. Ginger is a healing food that helps your immune and digestive systems.

For beef, the collagen in the bones breaks down into gelatin within about 48 hours, and for chicken it is about 24. You can make broth in less time, but to get the most out of the bones, I recommend making it in a crock pot closer to 48 hours.

Gelatin has amazing curative properties and even helps individuals with food sensitivities and allergies tolerate these foods more easily. It also promotes probiotic balance, while breaking down proteins making them easier to digest. The real truth about probiotics is that they help to create a healthy environment in your stomach.

During this first phase of the diverticulitis diet, consume only clear bone broths, clear fresh juices (no pulp), and soothing ginger tea.

Foods to Include and Exclude in the Clear Liquid Diet
During a diverticulitis flare-up, or at first symptoms, it is important to help your digestive tract clean itself out, and begin to heal. Start by using my beef bone broth recipe.

Eating bone broths made from beef, chicken, lamb and fish helps to heal leaky gut syndrome, improves joint health, boosts the immune system, and even helps to reduce cellulite, all while helping to heal the digestive tract.

Bone broths with cooked vegetables and a little bit of meat, provides essential nutrients your body needs, including calcium, magnesium, phosphorus, silicon, sulphur, and more, in an easily digested manner.

You may add vegetables to your bone broth including carrots, celery and garlic or for variation, you may add an egg poached in the broth. In addition, sip on warm ginger tea two to three times daily to help reduce inflammation and aid in digestion. Ginger is a healing food that helps your immune and digestive systems.

For beef, the collagen in the bones breaks down into gelatin within about 48 hours, and for chicken it is about 24. You can make broth in less time, but to get the most out of the bones, I recommend making it in a crock pot closer to 48 hours.

Gelatin has amazing curative properties and even helps individuals with food sensitivities and allergies tolerate these foods more easily. It also promotes probiotic balance, while breaking down proteins making them easier to digest. The real truth about probiotics is that they help to create a healthy environment in your stomach.

During this first phase of the diverticulitis diet, consume only clear bone broths, clear fresh juices (no pulp), and soothing ginger tea.

What to Avoid
During this first phase of the diverticulitis diet, consume only clear bone broths, clear fresh juices (no pulp), and soothing ginger tea.

Stage 2: The Juicing Diet

When your body has adapted to the foods in Stage 2, start to add fiber rich foods including raw fruits and vegetables, and unrefined grains, such as quinoa, black rice, fermented grains, or sprouted lentils. *It is important to stay away from whole nuts and seeds, as they can easily become trapped in the diverticula, causing further damage.*

According to researchers at the University of Oxford, fiber reduces the risk of diverticular disease. The study focused on fiber from fruits, vegetables, cereals, and potatoes.

Goals
According to researchers at the University of Oxford, fiber reduces the risk of diverticular disease. The study focused on fiber from fruits, vegetables, cereals, and potatoes.

Guidelines for the Juicing Diet
When your body has adapted to the foods in Stage 2, start to add fiber rich foods including raw fruits and vegetables, and unrefined grains, such as quinoa, black rice, fermented grains, or sprouted lentils. *It is important to stay away from whole nuts and seeds, as they can easily become trapped in the diverticula, causing further damage.*

Fruits to Include and Exclude in a Juicing Diet
When your body has adapted to the foods in Stage 2, start to add fiber rich foods including raw fruits and vegetables, and unrefined grains, such as quinoa, black rice, fermented grains, or sprouted lentils. *It is important to stay away from whole nuts and seeds, as they can easily become trapped in the diverticula, causing further damage.*

Vegetables to Include and Exclude in a Juicing Diet
When your body has adapted to the foods in Stage 2, start to add fiber rich foods including raw fruits and vegetables, and unrefined grains, such as quinoa, black rice, fermented grains, or sprouted lentils. *It is important to stay away from whole nuts and seeds, as they can easily become trapped in the diverticula, causing further damage.*

Stage 3: The Low Residue Diet

When your body has adapted to the foods in Stage 2, start to add fiber rich foods including raw fruits and vegetables, and unrefined grains, such as quinoa, black rice, fermented grains, or sprouted lentils. *It is important to stay away from whole nuts and seeds, as they can easily become trapped in the diverticula, causing further damage*

According to researchers at the University of Oxford, fiber reduces the risk of diverticular disease. The study focused on fiber from fruits, vegetables, cereals, and potatoes.

Goals
According to researchers at the University of Oxford, fiber reduces the risk of diverticular disease. The study focused on fiber from fruits, vegetables, cereals, and potatoes.

Guidelines
When your body has adapted to the foods in Stage 2, start to add

fiber rich foods including raw fruits and vegetables, and unrefined grains, such as quinoa, black rice, fermented grains, or sprouted lentils. *It is important to stay away from whole nuts and seeds, as they can easily become trapped in the diverticula, causing further damage.*

Stage 4: The High Fiber Diet

So over the first few days of stage four, introduce high-fiber foods gradually, adding just one new food every 3-4 days.

As your body starts to adapt you can begin consuming about 25-35 grams of fiber each day, to help stave off any potential flare-ups, while your digestive tract heals. Add in some potatoes, sweet potatoes, root vegetables, then slowly try some non-processed grains/beans such as oats or lentils.

One important distinction is the difference between soluble fiber, and insoluble fiber. Soluble fiber actually retains water, and turns into a gel during the digestive process. The gel helps to slow the digestion, allowing for greater absorption of essential nutrients. Insoluble fiber, on the other hand, adds bulk to stools, allowing foods to more quickly leave your system.

Foods high in soluble fiber include oat bran, nuts, seeds, beans, lentils barley, and peas. Insoluble fiber is found in foods including whole grains, wheat bran, and vegetables.

Researchers at the Department of Nutrition at Harvard Medical School found that it is the insoluble fiber that decreases risk for developing diverticular disease. But do not let this sway you from eating a balanced diet. You do not have to eliminate soluble fiber, nor should you.

Maintaining a healthy balance of protein, fiber, and fresh fruits and vegetables, is essential for keeping diverticulitis from flaring up.

Goals

As your body starts to adapt you can begin consuming about 25-35 grams of fiber each day, to help stave off any potential flare-ups, while your digestive tract heals. Add in some potatoes, sweet potatoes, root vegetables, then slowly try some non-processed grains/beans such as oats or lentils.

Guidelines

Maintaining a healthy balance of protein, fiber, and fresh fruits and vegetables, is essential for keeping diverticulitis from flaring up.

Foods to Include and Exclude in High Fiber Diet

Researchers at the Department of Nutrition at Harvard Medical School found that it is the insoluble fiber that decreases risk for developing diverticular disease. But do not let this sway you from eating a balanced diet. You do not have to eliminate soluble fiber, nor should you.

Foods to Completely Avoid in Diverticulitis Disease

Researchers at the Department of Nutrition at Harvard Medical School found that it is the insoluble fiber that decreases risk for developing diverticular disease. But do not let this sway you from eating a balanced diet. You do not have to eliminate soluble fiber, nor should you.

Fiber Contents of Foods (Including Market Products)

Fiber intake can be increased by eating whole-grain breads and cereals; fruits like apples and pears; vegetables like peas, spinach, and squash; and starchy vegetables like kidney and black beans.

THE 4 PHASE DIET RECIPES

JUICES PHASE 1

1. Devil's Juice
2. Carrot-Apple Smoothie
3. Coco-Turmeric Smoothie
4. Protein Smoothie
5. Protein Blueberry Smoothie
6. Bana-Berries Smoothie
7. Tea-Berries Smoothie
8. Plum-Yogurt Smoothie
9. Berry-Peach Frappuccino
10. Kiwi-Pineapple Frappuccino
11. Lemonade Berries Smoothie
12. Grape-Yogurt Frappuccino
13. Beet-Berries Smoothie
14. Apple-Beet Juice
15. Cucumber Juice
16. Dark Red Orange Juice
17. Apple-Pine Juice
18. Green Juice
19. Light Red Juice
20. Cherry-Walnut Smoothie
21. Fruity Frappuccino
22. Apple Spice Frappuccino
23. Pumpkin Spice Frappuccino

LOW RESIDUE PHASE 2

1. Baked Bacon Potato
2. Toast Sandwich
3. Quick-Baked Eggs
4. Bread-Onion Sauce
5. Cheesy Fish Sauce
6. Egg-Chicken Balls
7. Curry Chicken Sauce
8. Cheesy Soufflé
9. Creamy-Shredded Chicken
10. Creamy Fish Pie
11. Creamy Spaghetti
12. Healthy Potato Pie
13. Tomato-Potato Soup
14. Fish Soup
15. Vegan Pita Pizza
16. Cheesy Macaroni
17. Pasta-Ham Salad
18. Pavlova
19. Bana-Choco Bites
20. Crispy Sweet Potato Fries
21. Roasted Carrot Fries
22. Bonus Dipping

HIGH FIBER PHASE 3

1. Vegan Omelet
2. Roasted Lemon-Chicken
3. Lemon-Cauliflower Mashers
4. Sardine Salsa
5. Arugula Salad
6. Simple Vegan Salad
7. Blue cheese Mashers
8. Roasted Vegan-Beef
9. Veggie-Chicken Cobb Salad
10. Poached Green Salmon
11. Chickpeas & Steak
12. Beef Steak & Bok Choy
13. Wine-Mushroom Chicken
14. Omelet & Black Bean
15. Grilled Chicken & Citrus Salsa
16. Slow-Cooked Pork & Cabbage
17. White Bean Soup
18. Squid-Arugula Salad
19. Quinoa Pilaf
20. Yogurt-Chicken Soup
21. Miso Salmon Salad
22. Stir-Frying Veggies
23. Chicken Veggie Hot Pot
24. Thai Green Chicken Curry

BROTH PHASE 4

1. Slow-Cooked Beef Stew
2. Slit Peas & Veggie Soup
3. Hot Spice Squash Soup
4. Navy Veggie-Ham Soup
5. Tortellini Sausage Soup
6. Summer Vegan Soup
7. Barley-Chicken Soup
8. Time-Saving Condensed Soup
9. Fresh Veggie Soup
10. Creamy Chicken-Veggie Soup
11. Quick-Served Lentil Soup
12. Quick-Served Chicken Soup
13. Quick Chunky Soup
14. Turkey-Veggie Pie
15. Turkey-Veggie Soup
16. Thai Inspired Pumpkin Soup
17. Oven-Steamed Color Veggies
18. Rich Pumpkin Soup
19. Easy Sweet Potato Soup
20. Easy Zucchini Soup
21. Cheese-Chicken Rice Soup
22. Vegan-Bean Pasta
23. Deer-Corn Pie
24. Mother's Turkey Pasta
25. Vegan-Cashew Rice
26. Cream-Curry Vegan Soup
27. Cheesy Vegan Soup
28. Sherry Chicken Soup

JUICES

1. Devil's Juice

Ingredients
- 3 beets, cleaned and removed skin
- 5 celery stalks;
- 1 cup blueberries;
- 1 bunch of spinach leaves;
- 2 apples; washed, removed core and chopped
- 1 knuckle of ginger (or 2 teaspoon of minced fresh ginger)
- 1 knuckle of turmeric (or 2 teaspoon of minced fresh turmeric)
- 1 garlic clove; peeled

Directions

In juice maker, squeeze out juice from beet, celery, spinach leaves, apples, ginger, turmeric and blueberries. Mix together and serve in glass. ENJOY!

2. Carrot-Apple Smoothie

Ingredients
- 3 carrots; cleaned, removed skin if referred and chopped
- 2 green apple; washed, removed core and chopped
- 1/2 garlic clove; peeled
- 2 tablespoon lemon juice (about 1 lemon)
- 1 knuckle of ginger; washed and peeled

Directions
In blender, add carrot, green apple, lemon juice, ginger, garlic. Blend until smooth and creamy. Add ice if referred.
Serve in a glass. ENJOY!

3. Coco-Turmeric Smoothie

Ingredients
- 1 cup coconut oil (or hemp – your choice)
- ½ cup pineapple (or mango), bite-size cube and frozen
- 1 banana; peeled
- 1 tablespoon coconut oil
- ½ teaspoon turmeric powder (add more if referred)
- ½ teaspoon ginger powder
- 1 teaspoon chia seeds
- 1 teaspoon maca (optional)

Directions
In blender, add milk, banana, frozen pineapple, oil, turmeric, ginger, chia seeds and maca if used. Blend until smooth and creamy.
Serve in glass. ENJOY!

4. Protein Smoothie

Ingredients
- 1 cup mango cubes; frozen
- ½ cup sweet potato; cooked and chopped
- ½ cup pineapple juice
- 3/4 cup water
- 1 teaspoon cinnamon
- ½ teaspoon vanilla extract
- 1 teaspoon agave nectar (optional)

Directions

In blender, place sweet potato, mango, juice, cinnamon, water, vanilla and nectar if used. Blend until smooth and creamy.

Serve in glass and sprinkle cinnamon on top if desired. ENJOY!

5. Protein Blueberry Smoothie

Ingredients
- ½ cup soy protein milk (or your choice)
- 1 cup blueberries; frozen
- ¼ cup vanilla soy ice-cream (or yogurt – your choice)
- 1 banana; sliced and frozen
- 2 teaspoon rice protein powder
- 1 teaspoon chia seeds
- ½ tablespoon maple syrup (or honey – your choice)
- 1 teaspoon lemon juice (about ¼ lemon)

Directions

In blender, place ice-cream, milk, blueberries, banana, rice protein powder, chia seed, lemon juice and syrup. Blend until smooth and creamy.

Serve immediately in glass. ENJOY!

6. Bana-Berries Smoothie

Ingredients
- 1 small banana; peeled and frozen if referred
- 1 kiwi; removed skin and sliced
- ½ cup raspberries
- ½ tablespoon chia seeds
- 6 ice cubes (optional, use frozen fruit as ice)
- ½ cup water

Directions

In blender, add banana, kiwi, chia seed, raspberries, water and ice cubes. Blend until smooth and creamy.

Serve immediately in glass. ENJOY!

7. Tea-Berries Smoothie

Ingredients
- 6 oz Lipton pure green tea; brewed and chilled (2 bag of Lipton pure green tea, 6 oz hot water)
- 1 cup triple berry mix; frozen (or your choice of berry)
- ½ banana; sliced and frozen
- 1 ½ tablespoon honey (or maple syrup – your choice)
- 6 ice cubes (optional)

Directions

In blender, add chilled-brewed green tea, berry mix, banana and honey. Blend until smooth and creamy.

Serve immediately in glass with whip-topping on top if desired. ENJOY!

8. Plum-Yogurt Smoothie

Ingredients
- 5 oz low-fat Greek Yogurt;
- 1 cup blueberry; frozen
- 5 Prunes; dried (use Sun sweet Dried Prunes in this recipe)
- 8 oz Plum juice (use Sun sweet Light Plum Smart Juice in this recipe)
- 8 ice cubes (optional)

Directions

In blender, add yogurt, blueberry, prunes, juice and ice cubes. Blend until smooth and creamy.

Serve immediately in glass with whip-topping on top if desired. ENJOY!

9. Berry-Peach Frappuccino

Ingredients
- ¾ cup peaches; frozen
- ½ cup raspberries; frozen
- 1 teaspoon lemon juice (about ¼ lemon)
- ½ cup coconut milk (your choice of milk)
- 1 cup water
- ½ tablespoon chia seeds
- ½ tablespoon honey (or maple syrup – your choice)
- ¼ teaspoon vanilla extract

Directions

In blender, add peach, raspberries, lemon juice, milk, chia seed, honey, vanilla and water. Blend until smooth and creamy.

Serve immediately in glass with whip-topping on top if desired. ENJOY!

10. Kiwi-Pineapple Frappuccino

Ingredients
- 2 cup pineapple; chopped and frozen
- 2 kiwi; removed skin and cut into halves
- ½ cup pineapple juice (add more to reach your consistency)
- 2 tablespoon honey (or maple syrup – your choice)
- Ice cubes (optional)

Directions

In blender, add pineapple, kiwi, juice, honey and ice cubes if used. Blend until smooth and creamy.

Serve immediately in glass with whip-topping on top if desired. ENJOY!

11. Lemonade Berries Smoothie

Ingredients
- 1 cup lemonade (use Minute Maid 15 calorie Lemonade in this recipe)
- 1 cup mixed berries; frozen (or your choice of berry)

Directions

In blender, add berries and lemonade. Blend until smooth and creamy.

Serve immediately in glass with whip-topping on top if desired. ENJOY!

12. Grape-Yogurt Frappuccino

Ingredients
- 2 cup grape juice
- 1 cup blueberries; frozen
- 2 cup vanilla yogurt
- 6 ice cubes (optional)

Directions

In blender, add juice, blueberries, yogurt and ice cubes if used. Blend until smooth and creamy.

Serve immediately in glass with whip-topping on top if desired. ENJOY!

13. Beet-Berries Smoothie

Ingredients
- 9 carrots; cleaned, removed skin if needed and chopped
- 3 cup strawberries; washed and removed green part, chopped and frozen
- 1 cup blueberries; frozen
- 1 large beet; cleaned and chopped
- 1 knuckle ginger; fresh; peeled

Directions

In blender, add carrot, strawberries, blueberries, beet and ginger. Blend until smooth and creamy.

Serve immediately in glass with whip-topping on top if desired. ENJOY!

14. Apple-Beet Juice

Ingredients
- 1 beet; cleaned and peeled
- 1 apple; removed core
- 3 celery stalks
- 1 knuckle ginger; fresh; peeled

Directions

In juice maker, squeeze out and mix together juices of beet, apple, celery and ginger.

Serve immediately in glass. ENJOY!

15. Cucumber Juice

Ingredients
- 1 cucumber; cleaned
- 7 celery stalks
- 1 knuckle ginger; peeled
- 1 garlic clove; peeled

Directions

In juice maker, squeeze out and mix together juices of cucumber, garlic, celery and ginger.

Serve immediately in glass. ENJOY!

16. Dark Red Orange Juice

Ingredients
- 3 oranges; peeled and cut in halves
- 1 beet; removed skin and chopped
- 4 celery stalks;
- 1 cup spinach leaves; washed

Directions
In juice maker, squeeze out and mix together juices of beet, orange, celery, spinach.
Serve immediately in glass. ENJOY!

17. Apple-Pine Juice

Ingredients
- 2 green apples; removed cored and cut into quarters
- ¼ pineapple; chopped
- ½ cucumber; cleaned and cut into half

Directions

In juice maker, squeeze out and mix together juices of apple, pineapple and cucumber.

Serve immediately in glass. ENJOY!

18. Green Juice

Ingredients
- 2 green apples; removed cored and chopped
- 1 cup spinach leaves
- 1 Jicama (known as Mexican turnip); peeled and chopped
- 2 tablespoon key lime juice (about 1 key lime)

Directions

In juice maker, squeeze out and mix together juices of apple, spinach, and jicama and lime juice.

Serve immediately in glass. ENJOY!

19. Light Red Juice

Ingredients
- 2 carrots; cleaned, removed skin if referred and chopped
- 2 green apples; removed core and chopped
- 2 rhubarb stalks
- 2 teaspoon lemon juice (about ¼ lemon)
- 1 knuckle ginger; fresh, peeled

Directions

In juice maker, squeeze out and mix together juices of apple, carrot, rhubarb, lemon juice and ginger.

Serve immediately in glass. ENJOY!

20. Cherry-Walnut Smoothie

Ingredients
- 1 cup cherries; removed seed and frozen
- 1 cup strawberries; removed green part and cut into halves
- 1 cup kale
- 1/8 cup walnuts; chopped
- 1 teaspoon wheat germ
- ¾ cup green tea; brewed
- ½ teaspoon ginger; grated

Directions

In blender, add berries, cherries, kale, walnuts, wheat germ, green tea and lemonade. Blend until smooth and creamy.

Serve immediately in glass with whip-topping on top if desired. ENJOY!

21. Fruity Frappuccino

Ingredients
- 1 pear; removed skin, core and chopped
- 1 kiwi, peeled
- ¼ avocado
- 1 cup raspberries; frozen
- 1 cup spinach
- 3 oz non-fat vanilla Greek Yogurt
- ½ teaspoon flax seed meal
- 2 cup water; cold

Directions

In blender, add raspberries, spinach, kiwi, avocado, pear, yogurt, flax seed meal and water. Blend until smooth and creamy.

Serve immediately in glass with whip-topping on top if desired. ENJOY!

22. Apple Pie Frappuccino

Ingredients
- 1 apple (green or red – your choice); removed core and chopped
- ½ banana; chopped and frozen
- ½ cup almond milk; unsweetened (your choice of milk)
- ½ cup yogurt
- 1 tablespoon walnuts
- ¼ teaspoon cinnamon
- A pinch nutmeg
- 1 knuckle ginger; fresh; peeled and grated

Directions

In blender, add raspberries, spinach, kiwi, avocado, pear, yogurt, flax seed meal and water. Blend until smooth and creamy.

Serve immediately in glass with whip-topping on top if desired. ENJOY!

23. Pumpkin Spice Frappuccino

Ingredients
- ½ cup pumpkin puree; 100% pure, canned
- ½ banana; chopped and frozen
- ½ cup skim milk (or your choice of milk)
- ¼ teaspoon pumpkin spice mixture
- ½ brown sugar (or your choice of sweetener)
- ¼ teaspoon cinnamon
- ¼ teaspoon vanilla extract
- 6 ice cubes (optional)

Directions

In blender, add pumpkin puree, pumpkin spice, banana, milk, sugar, cinnamon and vanilla. Blend until smooth and creamy.

Serve immediately in glass with whip-topping and sprinkle cinnamon on top if desired. ENJOY!

LOW RESIDUE

1. Baked Bacon Potato

Ingredients
- 4 potatoes; cleaned and cut into halves
- 1 oz low-fat spread
- 8 bacon strips; chopped
- 4 tablespoon skim milk (or your choice)
- 4 oz low-fat cheddar cheese; shredded
- A dash of Worcestershire sauce
- Seasoning to taste: salt and pepper

Directions
1. Preheat oven to 400 degrees F.
2. Bake potato for 60 to 70 minutes or until tender. Set it aside for 10 minutes.
3. In skillet, on medium-high heat, cook and crumble bacon for 5 minutes. Remove from fat.
4. In mixing bowl, scoop out potato and mash with milk, 3 oz cheese, spread. Season with salt, pepper and sauce. Fold chopped bacon to incorporate.
5. Scoop into potato shell and sprinkle remaining cheese on top. Bake for 20 minutes or until melted cheese.
6. Serve immediately and sprinkle chopped fresh herb on top. ENJOY!

2. Toast Sandwich

Ingredients
- 8 oz Edam cheese; grated/ shredded (your choice)
- 4 eggs; Pasteur-raised
- 2 teaspoon flour
- 2 oz ham; cooked and chopped
- 4 slice of bread (use white bread in this recipe – your choice)
- A dash of Worcestershire sauce
- Seasoning to taste: salt and pepper

Directions
1. In mixing bowl, mix together egg, cheese, sauce and season with salt, pepper.
2. In skillet, on medium-high heat, toast one side of bread, about 2 minutes. Spread egg-cheese mixture on uncooked side and sprinkle with chopped ham then flip to cook, for 4 minutes more. Take out.
3. Serve bread with sprinkle more cheese on top if desired. ENJOY!

3. Quick-Baked Eggs

Ingredients
- 1 oz low-fat spread, melted
- 4 eggs; Pasteur-raised
- Seasoning to taste: salt and pepper

Directions
1. Preheat oven to 350 degrees F. grease ramekin with melt spread.
2. Crack each egg into separated ramekin. Bake for 5 to 8 minutes or until reach your flavor cooked egg. Sprinkle salt and pepper to taste.
3. Serve baked eggs with a slice of bread if desired. ENJOY!

4. Bread-Onion Sauce

Ingredients

- 3 slices of white bread
- 1 ½ cup skim milk (your choice)
- 1 onion; peeled and chopped
- 1 bay leaf
- 15 whole cloves (or grated nutmeg – your choice)
- 6 peppercorns
- 2 oz low-fat spread
- 2 tablespoon light double cream
- Seasoning to taste: salt and pepper

Directions

1. In food processor, blend white bread to make bread crumbs.
2. In saucepan, on medium heat, cook onion and grated nutmeg, about 3 minutes. Pour in milk and add bay leaf, peppercorn. Reduce to medium-low heat, cook for 15 to 25 minutes or until gently boiled.
3. Remove bay leaf, peppercorn and onion if referred.
4. Stir in bread crumb, spread and season with salt, pepper. Cook for 10 to 12 minutes or until swollen and sauce is thicken.
5. Serve hot/ warm sauce with baked chicken and sprinkle cooked onion on top if desired. ENJOY!

5. Cheesy Fish Sauce

Ingredients
- 1 pound white fish fillets; skinless and boneless
- 1 oz low-fat spread
- 1 oz white flour
- 1 cup skim milk; hot
- 1 ½ oz low-fat cheddar
- 8 oz potato; cooked and mashed
- Seasoning to taste: salt and pepper

Directions
1. In saucepan, on medium heat, bring milk to gently boil. Turn off heat, place fish fillet in hot milk, for 6 to 8 minutes. Drain and flake.
2. In other saucepan, on medium heat, melt spread and stir in flour, about 2 to 3 minutes. Gently pour milk and whisk constantly. Cook about 5 minutes. Stir in cheese and season with salt, pepper. Cook for 5 minutes more or until thicken.
3. Turn off heat and fold in fish until incorporated.
4. Serve fish sauce with cooked pasta or steam veggies if desired. ENJOY!

6. Egg-Chicken Balls

Ingredients
- 6 eggs; Pasteur-raised; hard-boiled, peeled and mashed
- 9 oz chicken; cooked and minced/ shredded
- 5 tablespoon low-fat mayonnaise
- 1 oz white bread crumbs
- Seasoning to taste: salt and pepper

Directions
1. In mixing bowl, mix mashed eggs, shredded chicken, mayonnaise and season with salt, pepper. Divide and shape into small balls.
2. Roll each small ball in bread crumbs until covered. Chilled at least 15 minutes.
3. Serve as snack or with rice and steamed veggies if desired. ENJOY!

7. Curry Chicken Sauce

Ingredients
- 4 chicken breasts; boneless and skinless
- 10 oz low-fat yogurt
- ½ teaspoon ginger powder
- ½ teaspoon paprika powder
- ½ tablespoon curry powder
- 2 tablespoon lemon juice (about 1 lemon)
- ½ teaspoon garlic powder
- Seasoning to taste: salt and pepper

Directions
1. Preheat oven to 325 degrees F.
2. In medium bowl, mix together yogurt, ginger, paprika, curry, lemon juice, garlic and season with salt, pepper.
3. In zip lock bag or shallow dish, pour yogurt-spice mixture over chicken breads or until covered. Refrigerate at least 6 hour or overnight.
4. Place chicken on rack over roasting tin. Pour yogurt-spice mixture on over chicken. Bake for 70 to 90 minutes or until cooked through.
5. Serve slice of chicken breast with rice or steamed veggies if desired. ENJOY!

8. Cheesy Soufflé

Ingredients
- 2 eggs; Pasteur-raised; separated egg white and egg yolk
- 1 teaspoon water
- ¼ oz low-fat spread
- Seasoning to taste: salt and pepper
- Low-fat cheese; grated (optional)

Directions
1. In mixing bowl, whisk egg white until soft peaks.
2. In medium bowl, whisk egg yolk with water until creamy. Gently fold in egg white to incorporate.
3. In omelet pan, on medium heat, melt spread and pour in egg batter. Cook for 2 to 4 minutes or until bottom is set and golden. Sprinkle grated cheese on top if used. Cook until melted cheese.
4. Serve immediately and fold in half if desired. ENJOY!

9. Creamy-Shredded Chicken

Ingredients
- 1 chicken; roasted and shredded meat
- 1 cup low-fat mayonnaise (add more if needed)
- 2 teaspoon curry powder
- 1 small onion; peeled and chopped
- ½ cup tomato juice
- ¼ cup red wine
- 3 tablespoon light cream
- 1 tablespoon apricot jam

Directions
1. In saucepan, on medium heat, brown onion with curry powder, about 3 minutes. Pour in red wine, tomato juice. Simmer for 10 to 15 minutes. Set it aside to cool down and chill.
2. In mixing bowl, add mayonnaise, apricot jam, low-fat cream and onion-liquid. Whisk to combine. Fold in shredded chicken to incorporate.
3. Serve creamy-shredded chicken with rice or steamed veggies if desired. ENJOY!

10. Creamy Fish Pie

Ingredients

- 1 pound fish (mix of haddock, cod and salmon – or your choice); skinless; rinsed and drained
- 1 ¾ cup skim milk (or your choice)
- 6 peppercorns
- 1 bay leaf
- 1 onion; peeled and cut into quarters
- 2 ½ oz low-fat spread
- 3 tablespoon white flour
- 2 eggs; Pasteur-raised; hard-boiled, peeled and chopped
- 1 egg; Pasteur-raised; lightly beaten
- 4 oz prawns; cooked
- 6 potatoes; peeled if referred, cooked and mashed

Directions

1. Preheat oven to 400 degrees F. grease baking pie pan with melt spread.
2. In saucepan, on medium heat, gently bring 1 cup milk with bay leaf, peppercorns, onion and salt. Turn off heat, place fish fillet in hot milk, for 6 to 8 minutes. Take out fish. Removed bay leaf, peppercorn, and onion. Strain cooking liquid.
3. In other saucepan, on medium heat, ½ oz melt spread and stir in flour, cook for 2 minutes. Cook with stirring in cooking liquid to prevent lump, for 6 to 8 minutes or until thicken. Turn off heat, stir in eggs, prawns and fish. Transfer into baking pie pan.
4. In mixing bowl, whisk mashed potato, milk, and remaining spread until incorporated. Spoon and spread over on top of meat-sauce. Bake for 10 to 15 minutes or until set. Brush beaten egg over and bake for 15 minutes more or until golden brown.
5. Serve a slice of pie with steamed veggies if desired. ENJOY!

11. Creamy Spaghetti

Ingredients
- 4 eggs; Pasteur-raised
- 5 oz single cream (low-fat)
- 8 oz bacon; chopped
- 12 oz spaghetti; cooked and drained
- 6 oz low-fat cheddar cheese; grated/ shredded
- Seasoning to taste: salt and pepper

Directions
1. In saucepan, on medium-high heat, cook bacon for 3 minutes or until crisp.
2. Reduce to medium-low heat, add cooked-drained spaghetti. Cook with stirring constantly to mix well. Add egg, 4 oz cheese, cream. Cook and stir well for 2 minutes. Turn off heat, keep stirring and egg will be cooked with remaining heat.
3. Serve immediately spaghetti and sprinkle remaining cheese on top with chopped parsley if desired. ENJOY!

12. Healthy Potato Pie

Ingredients
- 6 potatoes; cooked and mashed
- 2 teaspoon low-fat spread
- 2 large eggs; Pasteur-raised; lightly beaten
- 2 tablespoon skim milk (optional)
- 1 spring onion; chopped
- Seasoning to taste: salt and pepper
- Low-fat cheese; shredded

Directions
1. Preheat oven to 375 degrees F. grease well baking dish.
2. In food processor, place potato and add spread, milk, eggs, salt, and pepper. Blend until smooth or incorporated. Fold in chopped onion. Transfer into baking dish. Bake for 40 minutes or until lightly golden.
3. Serve potato pie and sprinkle with shredded cheddar cheese on top if desired. ENJOY!

13. Tomato-Potato Soup

Ingredients
- 1 large potato; peeled and sliced thinly
- 14 oz Tomato soup
- 1 tablespoon skim milk (add more if needed – your choice of milk)
- Seasoning to taste: salt and pepper

Directions
1. Preheat oven to 350 degrees F. Grease baking dish.
2. In mixing bowl, mix together tomato soup and skim milk to combine.
3. Place layer by layer potato into baking dish. Season with salt and pepper with each of layer potato. Pour tomato-milk over potato.
4. Cover with aluminum foil and bake for 60 to 80 minutes or until soften. Uncover and bake for 10 minutes more.
5. Serve with steamed fish or grilled steak if desired. ENJOY!

14. Fish Soup

Ingredients
- 1 pound haddock; fresh, skinless; cooked and flaked
- 1 cup tomato juice
- ½ cup skim milk (or your choice)
- 1 bay leaf
- 2 unsmoked bacon sliced; removed fat, chopped and cooked
- 2 garlic cloves; peeled and minced
- 2 potatoes; peeled and diced
- 1 cup fish stock
- Seasoning to taste: salt and pepper

Directions
1. In stock pot, on medium-high heat, add potatoes, tomato juice, stock, bay leaves, garlic, fish, bacon and season with salt, pepper. Bring to boil. Reduce to medium-low heat, simmer for 30 minutes with covered.
2. Uncover, remove bay leaf and stir in milk. Gently simmer for 10 minutes or until reheat.
3. Serve fish soup with steamed veggies or rice and bread if desired. ENJOY!

15. Vegan Pita Pizza

Ingredients
- 2 teaspoon olive oil (or your choice of oil)
- 1 teaspoon Italian seasoning mix ((substitute with mixture of dried herbs: basil, marjoram, oregano, rosemary, thyme and garlic)
- 1 teaspoon vinegar (use balsamic vinegar in this recipe, or your choice)
- 1 garlic cloves; peeled and minced
- 4 flat pita bread
- 2 tomatoes; sliced
- 1 cup low-fat mozzarella cheese; shredded
- 2 teaspoon basil leaves; fresh; chopped or snipped

Directions
1. Preheat oven to 425 degrees F. place parchment paper on baking sheet.
2. In small bowl, stir to combine oil, seasoning mix, vinegar and garlic.
3. In baking sheet, place pita bread separately. Brush one side of each pita bread with oil mixture. Sprinkle 2/3 cup cheese and tomato slice. Sprinkle remaining cheese on top.
4. Bake for 10 to 12 minutes or until melted cheese and lightly browned on the edges.
5. Serve immediately with sprinkle snipped fresh basil if desired. ENJOY!

16. Cheesy Macaroni

Ingredients

- 6 oz macaroni; cooked and drained
- 1 ½ oz low-fat spread
- 4 tablespoon white flour
- 2 cup skim milk (or your choice)
- 6 oz low-fat cheddar cheese; shredded
- 1 teaspoon nutmeg
- Seasoning to taste: salt and pepper

Directions

1. Preheat oven to 400 degrees F.
2. In saucepan, on medium heat, melt spread and stir in flour constantly to cook for a couple of minutes,
3. Reduce to medium-low heat, stir in milk and gently bring to boil. Cook for 6 to 8 minutes or until thicken. Turn off heat and season to taste with salt, pepper, nutmeg.
4. In baking dish, pour milk sauce over cheese and macaroni. Bake for 20 minutes or until golden and bubbling.
5. Serve cheesy macaroni with sprinkle bread crumbs on top if desired. ENJOY!

17. Pasta-Ham Salad

Ingredients
- 8 oz pasta (your choice); cooked and drained
- 4 oz ham; sliced or diced
- 1 oz parmesan cheese; grated
- ½ cup low-fat dressing for salad
- 4 oz mushroom; cleaned and sliced
- 1 teaspoon low-fat spread
- 1 garlic clove; peeled and diced

Directions
1. In saucepan, on medium heat, melt spread. Cook and brown mushroom and garlic for 3 to 5 minutes.
2. In large bowl, add ham, salad dressing, parmesan cheese and cooked mushroom. Fold to toss well. Then place cooked pasta and toss until dressing cover pasta.
3. Serve pasta-ham and sprinkle cheese and white bread crumbs on top if desired. ENJOY!

18. Pavlova

Ingredients
- 1 cup caster sugar
- 1 teaspoon cornstarch
- 3 egg whites; Pasteur-raised, room-temperature
- 1 teaspoon vinegar
- 1 teaspoon vanilla extract

Directions
1. Preheat oven 300 degrees F. place parchment paper on baking sheet.
2. In mixing bowl, whisk egg white with sugar until soft peaks. Whisk gently corn starch, vanilla, vinegar in egg whites until smooth and stiff peaks.
3. Transfer and shape into a circle. Bake at 275 degrees F for 1 hours or until dry and crisp. Let it cool down inside oven about 1 hour or overnight.
4. Serve Pavlova with a spoon of whip-topping or ice-cream if desired. ENJOY!

19. Bana-Choco Bites

Ingredients
- 1 banana; peeled, sliced and frozen at least 1 hour
- 1 cup chocolate chips (your choice of dark/ milk)
- 1 tablespoon coconut oil (or butter; grass-fed – your choice)
- ¼ cup peanut butter

Directions
1. In microwave, melt chocolate chip and oil, for 30 seconds. Stir in peanut butter until smooth and let cool slightly.
2. Dip each of frozen banana in Choco-peanut mix until cover and place in parchment paper. Freeze until firm.
3. Serve immediately after take out of freezer. ENJOY!

20. Crispy Sweet Potato Fries

Ingredients
- 2 medium sweet potatoes; peeled and cut into long sticks
- 2 tablespoon olive oil
- 1 teaspoon paprika powder (optional)
- Seasoning to taste: salt and pepper

Directions
1. Preheat oven to 425 degrees F. place aluminum foil on baking sheet.
2. In large bowl, toss to cover well carrot sticks with oil, salt, pepper and paprika powder if used.
3. Spread into baking sheet and bake for 15 minutes. Flip and bake for 10 to 15 minutes more or until caramelized and crispy.
4. Serve with your flavor dipping if desired. ENJOY!

21. Roasted Carrot Fries

Ingredients
- 2 pound carrots (or mini carrot; your choice); cleaned, removed skin if referred and cut into long stick
- 2 tablespoon olive oil
- 2 teaspoon thyme leaves; chopped
- Seasoning to taste: salt and pepper

Directions
1. Preheat oven to 425 degrees F. place aluminum foil on baking sheet.
2. In large bowl, toss to cover well carrot sticks with oil, salt, pepper, thyme.
3. Spread into baking sheet and bake for 20 to 25 minutes or until caramelized and tender.
4. Serve with your flavor dipping if desired. ENJOY!

22. Bonus Dipping

Ingredients
- ½ cup peanut butter
- ½ cup vanilla Greek Yogurt
- ¼ teaspoon cinnamon
- 2 tablespoon chocolate chip (optional)
- 2 teaspoon honey (or your choice of sweetener)

Directions
1. In mixing bowl, mix together peanut butter, yogurt, cinnamon and honey. Fold in chocolate chips if used. Refrigerate to chill.
2. Serve yogurt-butter dipping with fresh fruit or pretzels if desired. ENJOY!

HIGH FIBER

1. Vegan Omelet

Ingredients
- ½ small tomato; chopped
- 2 teaspoon olive oil
- 8 large egg whites; Pasteur-raised
- ½ small onion; peeled and chopped
- 2 cup spinach leaves; fresh
- 1 tablespoon water
- Seasoning to taste: salt and pepper

Directions
1. In skillet, on medium heat, cook onion with oil until translucent, about 3 minutes. Stir in tomatoes, spinach leaves and season with salt, pepper. Cook for 3 minutes more. Transfer to bowl and cover to keep warm.
2. Meanwhile, in medium bowl, whisk egg white with water and a pinch of salt until frothy.
3. In nonstick skillet or omelet pan, on medium heat, add egg white and swirl to cover pan. Cook for 2 to 3 minutes or until set then flip.
4. Serve egg white with a spoon of tomato-spinach then fold into half and sprinkle more chopped parsley on top if desired. ENJOY!

2. Roasted Lemon-Chicken

Ingredients
- 2 tablespoon olive oil
- 10 Kalamata olives; cut into halves
- 4 oz feta cheese; crumbled
- 4 tablespoon lemon juice (about 2 lemon)
- 2 lemon; sliced
- 2 chicken breast; pasture-raised; skin-in and boneless
- 4 garlic cloves; peeled and chopped
- 1 tablespoon mint leaves; fresh, chopped
- 1 tablespoon oregano; fresh, chopped
- Seasoning to taste: salt and pepper

Directions
1. Preheat oven to 350 degrees F.
2. Rub garlic between skin and meat of chicken. Toss to cover chicken with oil, lemon juice and sprinkle salt, pepper to taste.
3. Place a single layer of sliced lemon on bottom of baking dish. Transfer chicken on layer of lemon and sprinkle chopped mint-oregano on top.
4. Cover with aluminum oil or lid on and bake for 40 minutes, until juice run clear. Uncover, sprinkle feta cheese on over and bake for 5 minutes more.
5. Serve immediately with oregano and mint on top if desired. ENJOY!

3. Lemon-Cauliflower Mashers

Ingredients
- ¼ cup buttermilk; grass-fed
- 4 cup cauliflowers; chopped
- 1/3 cup parsley; fresh, chopped
- 1 tablespoon lemon juice (about half of lemon)
- 1 tablespoon butter; grass-fed
- Seasoning to taste: salt and pepper

Directions
1. In microwave or steamer, steam cauliflower until soft.
2. In food processor, add cauliflower, buttermilk, butter, lemon juice, 1/6 cup parsley, salt and pepper. Blend until smooth. Fold in remaining parsley.
3. Serve with grilled steak if desired. ENJOY!

4. Sardine Salsa

Ingredients
- 2 tins (about 4.375 oz/ tin) Wild Planet Sardines
- 6 tablespoon olive oil
- 16 black olives, cut into halves
- 8 cup lettuces (or your choice); chopped
- 2 cup green beans; cut into bite-sized long
- 4 tablespoon vinegar (use red wine vinegar in this recipe – or your choice)
- 16 grape tomatoes
- 1 small onion; peeled and sliced thinly
- 2 teaspoon Dijon mustard
- 2 large eggs; Pasteur-raised; hard-boiled, peeled and sliced
- Seasoning to taste: salt and pepper

Directions
1. In saucepan, on medium-high heat, cook green beans for 3 minutes or until crispy.
2. In large bowl, whisk together vinegar, mustard, oil, salt and pepper until lightly thicken.
3. Serve in a salad bowl or plate with lettuce, sliced eggs, sardines, tomatoes, green beans, onion, and olives and drizzle dressing over. ENJOY!

5. Arugula Salad

Ingredients
- 2 tablespoon olive oil
- 1 teaspoon honey (or maple syrup – your choice)
- 1 avocado; ripe; removed skin, seed and sliced
- 4 medium radishes; cleaned and sliced thinly
- 1 small onion; peeled and sliced thinly
- 6 cup Arugula; fresh; rinsed
- 2 tablespoon balsamic vinegar
- 2 cans (about 6 oz/ can) Salmon (use brand of Wild Planet Alaskan Sockeye Salmon in this recipe); drained and flaked
- 1 medium tomato; washed and cut into chunks
- Seasoning to taste: salt and pepper

Directions
1. In small bowl, whisk oil, vinegar, honey, salt and pepper until lightly thicken.
2. In serving bowl, place arugula, avocado, onion, radishes, tomato, and salmon and drizzle dressing over. Toss if desired. ENJOY!

6. Simple Vegan Salad

Ingredients
- 1 teaspoon olive oil; extra-virgin
- 3 tablespoon lemon juice (about 1 ½ lemon)
- 1 ½ cup cherry tomatoes, cut into halves
- 6 cup lettuce; shredded or chopped
- 8 Kalamata olives; sliced
- 2 scallions; peeled and sliced
- 1 tablespoon parsley leaves; fresh, chopped
- 2 garlic cloves; peeled and minced
- 2 oz feta cheese; crumbled
- ¾ teaspoon dried oregano
- Seasoning to taste: salt and pepper

Directions
1. In small bowl, whisk together oil, lemon juice, oregano, garlic, salt and pepper until lightly thicken.
2. In large bowl, place lettuce, scallion, tomato, olives and pour dressing over. Toss gently to combine.
3. Serve salad with more dressing and feta cheese on top if desired. ENJOY!

7. Blue-cheese Mashers

Ingredients
- 3 oz blue cheese; grass-fed
- 2 head of cauliflowers; cut into bite-size pieces
- 2 tablespoon chives; fresh; chopped
- 2 teaspoon paprika powder
- Seasoning to taste: salt and pepper

Directions
1. In steamer or saucepan, cook or steam cauliflower until soft. Drain and cool slightly.
2. In food processor, blend cauliflower and season with salt, pepper, paprika powder until creamy or reach your consistency. Fold in blue cheese and fresh chives.
3. Serve cheese-mashers with steamed veggies or grilled steak if desired. ENJOY!

8. Roasted Vegan-Beef

Ingredients
- 12 oz Beef Roast
- 2 large sweet potatoes; washed and cooked
- 2 cup broccoli; washed, cut into bite-sized pieces and steamed
- 4 teaspoon almond; sliced and toasted
- 1 onion; peeled and sliced
- 1 tablespoon lemon juice (about ½ lemon)
- Seasoning to taste: salt and pepper

Directions
1. Preheat oven to 400 degrees F.
2. In saucepan, on high heat, brown each side of beef, about 3 minutes. Transfer into baking dish and bake for 50 to 60 minutes.
3. In same saucepan, on medium-high heat, brown onion, broccoli, sweet potatoes and almond with lemon juice, salt, pepper to taste. Cook for 2 minutes.
4. Serve slice of beef, veggies and sprinkle chopped fresh herbs on top if desired. ENJOY!

9. Veggie-Chicken Cobb Salad

Ingredients
- 2 chicken breast; Pasteur-raised, skinless and boneless
- 1 avocado; removed skin, seed and diced
- 1 cucumber; peeled if referred and sliced
- 4 eggs; Pasteur-raised; hard-boiled, peeled and sliced
- 10 cup lettuce; fresh, organic; rinsed and chopped if referred
- 20 grape tomatoes; washed and drained
- ¼ cup blue cheese; crumbled
- Seasoning to taste: salt and pepper

Directions
1. In saucepan, on medium-high heat, cook chicken with water. Bring to boil, about 3 minutes. Reduce to medium heat, simmer with covered for 10 minutes. Turn off heat and let it cook in remaining hot water for 10 minutes more. Drain and slice.
2. Serve chicken, veggies with blue cheese and flavor dressing on top if desired. ENJOY!

10. Poached Green Salmon

Ingredients
- 3 tomatoes; chopped roughly
- 1 tablespoon parsley; chopped
- 1 cup white wine
- ½ cup water
- 2 tablespoon olive oil
- 8 oz spinach; fresh
- 1 medium onion; peeled and chopped
- 16 oz salmon; skinless, boneless
- Seasoning to taste: salt and pepper

Directions
1. In saucepan, on medium-high heat, bring wine, water to boil. Reduce to medium-low heat, place salmon. Simmer with covered for 6 to 8 minutes. Drain and flake salmon.
2. In skillet, on medium-high heat, brown onion and tomato with oil, for 4 to 6 minutes or until onions are translucent.
3. Serve salmon on lettuce with browned tomato-onion and sprinkle parsley on top if desired. ENJOY!

11. Chickpeas & Steak

Ingredients
- ½ cilantro; chopped
- 2 oz feta cheese; grass-fed
- 1 tablespoon oil (or your choice of oil)
- 8 cup mixed baby greens
- 1 cup chick Peas; rinsed and drained
- 24 oz strip steak; grass-fed
- 2 tablespoon lemon juice (about 1 lemon)
- 1 tomato; chopped
- Seasoning to taste: salt and pepper

Directions
1. In skillet, on medium-high heat, heat oil and cook steak, about 4 to 6 minutes per side. Set it aside to cool at least 5 minutes before slicing.
2. In same skillet, on medium-high heat, cook with stirring chick peas, about 3 to 5 minutes or until crispy. Add in tomatoes, cilantro, lemon juice and season with salt, pepper to taste. Cook and stir constantly about 3 minutes or heat through.
3. Serve sliced steak with chickpea mixture and sprinkle feta cheese on top. ENJOY!

12. Beef Steak & Bok Choy

Ingredients
- 4 heads of bok choy; chopped
- 2 tablespoon vinegar (your choice of vinegar)
- ¼ cup water
- 1 pound beef steak; grass-fed
- 1 tablespoon oil (your choice)
- 2 tablespoon gluten-free soy sauce / tamari
- 1 tablespoon ginger; fresh, peeled and grated
- 1 teaspoon stevia (or your choice of sweetener)
- Seasoning to taste: salt and pepper

Directions
1. In skillet, on medium-high heat, heat oil, cook steak and season with salt, pepper, about 4 to 6 minutes per side. Set it aside.
2. In saucepan, on medium-high heat, add bok choy, water. Cook with covered for 2 to 3 minutes or until tender.
3. Uncover and stir in soy sauce, vinegar, ginger and stevia. Bring to boil. Add steak and toss for 1 to 2 minutes more.
4. Serve sliced steak with bok choy and remaining juices on top. ENJOY!

13. Wine-Mushroom Chicken

Ingredients
- 1 bell pepper; cleaned, removed seed and chopped
- 16 oz button mushroom; cleaned and cut into quarters
- 2 garlic cloves; peeled and minced
- 8 cup spinach leaves; rinsed and drained
- ½ cup dry white wine
- 2 tablespoon avocado oil (or your choice)
- 3 chicken breast; boneless, skinless and Pasteur-raised
- Seasoning to taste: salt and pepper

Directions
1. In skillet, on medium-high heat, cook chicken with oil, for 5 to 7 minutes each side or until golden brown. Set it aside.
2. In same skillet, on medium-high heat, cook and stir mushroom, bell pepper with remaining oil, for 3 minutes. Add garlic and wine. Cook for 2 to 3 minutes or until mushroom tender. Turn off heat, toss in spinach and season with salt, pepper to taste.
3. Serve mushroom-pepper and sauce over chicken. ENJOY!

14. Omelet & Black Bean

Ingredients
- 2 oz cheddar cheese; shredded
- 1 tablespoon cilantro; fresh; chopped
- 2 teaspoon avocado oil
- 4 large eggs; Pasteur-raised
- ¼ teaspoon chili powder
- ½ cup Black beans
- Seasoning to taste: salt and pepper

Directions
1. In medium bowl, whisk together eggs, chili powder, and salt and pepper until frosty.
2. In skillet, on medium-high heat, heat oil. Pour egg mixture and swirl to evenly coat. Sprinkle black bean, cheese and cilantro on top. Cook with covered for 2 minutes or until melted cheese.
3. Serve immediately with steamed veggies if desired. ENJOY!

15. Grilled Chicken & Citrus Salsa

Ingredients
- 8 chicken drumsticks; Pasteur-raised
- 2 scallions; peeled and chopped
- 2 tablespoon lime juices;
- 1 lime; cut into wedges
- 1 cup red grapefruit juices (about 1 fruit)
- 1 cup red grapefruit sections (about 1 fruit)
- 2 tablespoon mint leaves; fresh; chopped
- 2 tablespoon cilantro; fresh; chopped
- ¼ cup olive oil
- Seasoning to taste: salt and pepper

Directions
1. Preheat grill on medium-high heat.
2. In large bowl, stir to combine 1 teaspoon oil, lime juice, red grapefruit juice, 1 tablespoon cilantro, 1 tablespoon mint, salt and pepper. Place chicken in mixture and toss to cover. Set it aside for at least 30 minutes to 4 hours.
3. Grill and turn chicken occasionally on medium-high heat for 8 to 10 minutes or until cook through.
4. Meanwhile, in medium bowl, toss gently grapefruit sections, scallion with remaining oil, cilantro and mint. Season to taste with salt, pepper.
5. Serve grilled chicken with citrus salsa and lime wedges if desired. ENJOY!

16. Slow-Cooked Pork & Cabbage

Ingredients
- 2 tablespoon coconut oil (or your choice)
- 1 large onion; peeled and chopped
- 2 garlic cloves; peeled and minced
- 1 tablespoon honey
- 36 oz Tenderloin pork
- ½ cup apple cider vinegar (or your choice of vinegar)
- 1 head of green cabbage; washed and cut into 8 wedges
- ½ teaspoon thyme; dried
- Seasoning to taste: salt and pepper

Directions
1. Preheat oven to 325 degrees F.
2. In small bowl, stir to combine vinegar, honey, garlic.
3. In skillet, on medium-high heat, melt oil. Brown onion, pork and season with salt, pepper. Transfer into baking dish.
4. Place cabbage around pork and pour over vinegar-honey mixture. Cover with aluminum foil. Bake for 3 hours or until internal pork temperature reach 160 degrees F.
5. Serve pork and cabbages immediately if desired. ENJOY!

17. White Bean Soup

Ingredients
- 1 can (about 16 oz) northern beans; rinsed and drained
- 1 tablespoon dried rosemary
- 4 cup chicken broth (or your choice of broth)
- 6 garlic cloves; peeled and minced
- 1 medium onion; peeled and chopped
- 2 tablespoon olive oil
- ½ cup sun-dried tomatoes
- Seasoning to taste: salt and pepper

Directions
1. In stock pot, on medium heat, add oil and brown onion, garlic for 3 to 4 minutes. Add broth, rosemary, beans, tomatoes and season with salt, pepper. Simmer for 15 minutes or until reach your flavor consistency.
2. Serve warm soup with grilled steak if desired. ENJOY!

18. Squid-Arugula Salad

Ingredients
- 1/3 cup olive oil
- 16 oz squid; cut and separated bodies and tentacles into bite-size
- 1 ½ cup cherry tomatoes; cut into halves
- 6 cup baby arugula; washed
- 1 can (about 16 oz) white beans; rinsed and drained
- 3 tablespoon lemon juices (about 1 ½ lemon)
- Seasoning to taste: salt and pepper

Directions
1. In saucepan or steamer, steam squid for 3 minutes or until tender. Set it aside.
2. In large bowl, place arugula, tomatoes, beans, squid, oil, juice and season with salt, pepper. Toss to cover evenly.
3. Serve with a slice of bread if desired. ENJOY!

19. Quinoa Pilaf

Ingredients
- 6.5 oz artichokes in water
- 1 tomatoes; washed and diced
- 2 cup vegetable broth (or your choice)
- 1 tablespoon olive oil
- 8 Kalamata olives; cut into halves
- ½ teaspoon garlic powder
- 1 cup quinoa; rinsed
- 1 scallion; peeled and diced
- 1 teaspoon lemon zest (about ¼ lemon)
- Seasoning to taste: salt and pepper

Directions
1. In saucepan, on medium heat, combine quinoa, garlic, lemon zest, oil, salt, pepper and broth. Simmer with covered, about 15 to 20 minutes or until quinoa absorbed liquid. Turn off heat and stir in tomato, artichokes, scallion, and olives to combine.
2. Serve warm pilaf with garnish chopped parsley on top if desired. ENJOY!

20. Yogurt-Chicken Soup

Ingredients
- 1 tablespoon coconut oil
- 2 bell peppers; removed seed and sliced thinly
- 1 onion; peeled and sliced thinly
- 3 tablespoon paprika powder
- ½ cup dry white wine
- 1 tablespoon lemon juice (about ½ lemon)
- ½ cup chicken broth (or your choice)
- 1 can (about 28 oz) tomatoes with basil
- ¼ cup Greek yogurt
- 2 tablespoon parsley leaves; fresh; chopped
- 4 chicken breasts; boneless, skinless and Pasteur-raised
- Seasoning to taste: salt and pepper

Directions
1. In saucepan, on medium-high heat, melt oil. Brown and season each side of chicken for 3 minutes or until golden. Set it aside.
2. In same saucepan, on medium-high heat, brown onion, bell pepper until onion translucent, about 5 minutes. Stir in paprika, wine, broth, lemon juice, tomatoes. Bring to boil. Reduce to medium-low heat, place in chicken and simmer with cover for 8 to 10 minutes or until cooked through chicken. Turn off heat, stir in yogurt until incorporated.
3. Serve immediately with chopped fresh parsley on top if desired. ENJOY!

21. Miso Salmon Salad

Ingredients
- 4 tablespoon olive oil
- 1 cup baby spinach; washed and drained
- 1 ½ tablespoon brown rice Miso
- 1 ½ teaspoon tamari – gluten-free soy sauce
- ½ teaspoon sesame oil
- 24 oz salmon; skinless
- 6 tablespoon lemon juice (about 3 lemons)
- 2 tablespoon ginger; fresh; peeled and grated
- 2 tablespoon chives; chopped
- Seasoning to taste: salt and pepper

Directions
1. In medium bowl; stir together ¾ tablespoon miso, 2 tablespoon lemon juice, and 1 tablespoon ginger and sesame oil. Add salmon and toss gently to coat. Set aside at least 10 minutes.
2. In skillet, on medium-high heat, place and cook salmon, about 6 to 8 minutes or until cook outside but still pink inside.
3. Meanwhile, in small bowl, mix remaining of miso, ginger, lemon juice, chives and soy sauce, oil salt, pepper.
4. Serve cooked salmon, spinach and drizzle vinaigrette over on top. ENJOY!

22. Stir-Frying Veggies

Ingredients
- 2 zucchini; cleaned and sliced
- 1 bell pepper; removed seed and sliced
- 1 small onion; peeled and sliced
- 1 cup shitake mushroom;
- 2 teaspoon sesame oil
- ½ tablespoon tamari – gluten-free soy sauce

Directions
1. In skillet, on medium-high heat, brown onion with oil for 2 minutes. Add mushroom, tamari to cook with stirring for 3 minutes. Add bell pepper, zucchini and cook with stirring for 3 to 5 minutes or until crispy and tender.
2. Serve veggies with a bed of rice if desired. ENJOY!

23. Chicken Veggie Hot Pot

Ingredients
- 20 shitake mushrooms; fresh, organic
- 3 cup bok choy; sliced
- 4 cup low-sodium chicken broth
- 4 teaspoon vinegar (use rice vinegar in this recipe, or your choice of vinegar)
- 1 tablespoon fish sauce
- 1 cup water
- 3 tablespoon ginger; peeled and chopped
- 3 tablespoon gluten-free soy sauce (tamari)
- 3 teaspoon sesame oil
- 4 chicken breasts; boneless and skinless, Pasteur-raised
- 2 green onion; sliced
- Seasoning to taste: salt and pepper

Directions
1. In saucepan, on medium-high heat, cook chicken with water. Bring to boil, about 3 minutes. Reduce to medium heat, simmer with covered for 10 minutes. Turn off heat and let it cook in remaining hot water for 10 minutes more. Drain and shredded.
2. In stock pot, on medium-high heat, pour broth, water, mushroom and ginger. Bring to boil. Reduce to medium heat, stir in fish sauce, soy sauce, sesame oil and simmer for 3 to 5 minutes. Add shredded chicken, bok choy and vinegar. Simmer for 2 minutes or until choy is tender. Season to taste with salt, pepper.
3. Serve warm/ hot chicken soup with green onion on top. ENJOY!

24. Thai Green Chicken Curry

Ingredients

- 2 Chicken breast; boneless, skinless; cut into bite-sized pieces
- 1 cup Rice noodle; cooked and drained
- 1 Potatoes; cleaned, peeled if needed and cut into quarter
- 1 Carrots; cleaned, peeled if needed and chopped
- 1 medium eggplants; washed and chopped into bite-sized pieces
- 1 scallion; peeled and sliced
- 1 cup coconut cream
- 1 cup chicken stock
- 2 teaspoon curry paste
- 1 tablespoon olive oil
- Seasoning to taste: salt and pepper

Directions

1. In saucepan, on medium-high heat, brown potato, carrot and chicken with oil for 4 minutes. Stir in eggplant, scallion and cook for 5 minutes more. Pour coconut cream, curry paste, chicken stock. Reduce to medium heat, bring to boil gently for 10 to 15 minutes or until tender vegetables and cooked chicken. Season to taste with salt, pepper.
2. Serve warm curry chicken-veggies over rice noodle with sprinkle chopped chives on top if desired. ENJOY!

BROTH

1. Slow-Cooked Beef Stew

Ingredients
- 3 pound beef chuck roast; boneless;
- 6 medium potatoes; washed and cut into quarter
- 2 carrots; washed and cut into bite-size
- 2 cup mushroom; fresh; cleaned and removed stems if needed
- 2 small yellow onion; peeled and sliced
- 1 packet of Lipton Onion Soup dry mix (or substitute with onion flakes, low-sodium beef granules, onion powder, parsley flakes, celery seed; paprika powder and pepper)
- 1 cup broth (or your choice of broth; use beef broth to add more flavor in this recipe)
- 1 tablespoon butter; grass-fed (or your choice of fat/ oil; optional)

Directions
1. In skillet, on medium-high heat, melt butter and brown beef, about 3 minutes each side of meat. Set it aside.
2. In crock pot, stir to dissolve soup mix in broth. Add carrot, onion, potatoes, mushroom, and browned beef. Cook on low for 8 to 9 hours.
3. Serve beef-veggie stew with a bed of rice if desired. ENJOY!

2. Slit Peas & Veggie Soup

Ingredients
- 1 cup yellow slit peas; rinsed and drained
- 5 cup waters
- 2 ½ teaspoon (about 2 ½ cubes) vegetable bouillon; gluten free
- 2 large carrots; peeled if needed and chopped
- 2 celery stalks; chopped
- 1 yellow onion; peeled and chopped
- 1 large potato; cleaned skin well and chopped
- 1 bay leaf
- Seasoning to taste: salt and pepper

Directions
1. In large soup pot, on high heat, bring water to boil. Add bouillon and stir to dissolve. Add carrots, potatoes, onion, slit pea and bay leaf. Reduce to low heat, cook with covered and stir frequently, about 90 minutes or until thicken. Uncover and season with salt, pepper to taste. Remove bay leaf.
2. Serve warm with slice of wheat bread or a bed of rice if desired. ENJOY!

3. Hot Spice Squash Soup

Ingredients
- 1 butternut squash; removed seed, skin and chopped
- 1 garlic clove; peeled and minced
- 1 small potato; cleaned, peeled if needed and cut into half
- 1 parsnip; cleaned and cut into quarter
- 1 yellow onion; peeled and sliced
- 1/3 cup carrot; chopped
- 2 teaspoon ginger; fresh; minced
- 2 cup stock (or your choice; or use chicken stock as this recipe)
- 1 teaspoon garam masala (or substitute with mixture of ground spice: cinnamon, cumin, cardamom, cloves, peppercorn)
- 2 tablespoon olive oil
- Seasoning to taste: salt and pepper

Directions
1. Preheat oven to 300 degrees F. place parchment on baking sheet.
2. Toss to cover squash, parsnip, potato with 1 ½ tablespoon oil, ginger and garlic. Spread into baking sheet. Bake for an hour.
3. Meanwhile, in large soup pot, on medium-high heat, toss and cook carrot, onion with remaining oil, about 3 minutes or until brown and soft.
4. Reduce on medium-low heat, add stock, roasted vegetables and season with salt, pepper, garam masala. Simmer with covered about 1 hour. Blend until smooth with hand mixer.
5. Serve hot/ warm with sprinkle cinnamon on top if desired. ENJOY!

4. Navy Veggie-Beef Soup

Ingredients
- 1 pound ground beef; grass-feed
- 5 small potatoes; cleaned and peeled if referred
- 2 celery stalks; chopped
- 1 cup baby carrot; cleaned
- ½ package of Frozen mixed Vegetables
- 32 oz broth (vegetable/ chicken/ beef broth – your choice)
- 1 package (about 2 teaspoon or 1 cube) Lipton 'Onion Soup Mix
- 1 can (about 28 oz.) diced tomatoes; drained
- 1 can (about 16 oz.) navy beans; drained
- 4 bacon strips; chopped
- Seasoning to taste: salt and pepper

Directions
1. In skillet, on medium-high heat, cooked bacon until crumble. Take out.
2. In same skillet, on high heat, add ground beef into bacon fat and season to taste with salt, pepper. Cook until brown.
3. In crock pot, add celery, carrot, potato, garlic, broth, Lipton' Onion Soup Mix, navy beans, frozen vegetables and brown beef. Cook on low for 8 to 10 hours or on high for 4 to 6 hour.
4. Serve warm veggie-beef soup with 1 cup of cooked Pasta or rice and sprinkle cooked-crumble bacon on top if desired. ENJOY!

5. Tortellini Sausage Soup

Ingredients
- 1 pound Italian sausage; removed cased and sliced
- 1 teaspoon olive oil (optional)
- 1 yellow onion; peeled and chopped
- 1 can (about 28 oz.) diced tomatoes, drained
- 2 carrots; peeled and sliced
- 1 large summer squash; washed and sliced
- 1 green pepper; removed seed and chopped
- 2 garlic cloves; peeled and minced
- 1 can (about 14.5 oz) beef broth (or your choice of broth)
- 1 teaspoon dried basil
- 1 teaspoon dried oregano
- A bunch of parsley; chopped (about 3 tablespoon)
- 1 box (about 7 oz.) Tortellini Cheese
- ½ cup Parmesan cheese; grated
- Seasoning to taste: salt and pepper

Directions
1. In frying pan, on medium heat, cook sausage with oil for 10 to 12 minutes.
2. In stockpot, on medium-low heat, add sausage, tomato, carrot, squash, green pepper, basil, oregano, parsley, garlic, onion, broth and water if needed to cover everything. Cook with covered for 40 to 60 minutes or until vegetables are tender.
3. Uncovered and add tortellini cheese. Cook for 10 minutes more or until tender.
4. Serve hot with grated parmesan cheese on top. ENJOY!

6. Summer Vegan Soup

Ingredients
- 8 cup vegetable broth (your choice of broth)
- 4 carrots; removed skin if referred and sliced (about 2 cup)
- 5 to 6 celery stalks; cleaned and sliced
- 1 large yellow squash; cleaned and sliced
- 1 large zucchini; fresh; cleaned and sliced
- 2 tomatoes; washed and chopped
- 1 large yellow onion; peeled and chopped
- 1 pound kidney beans; dark-red beans; rinsed and soaked overnight (or at least 6 hours before cook)
- ½ cabbage; washed and chopped (about 2 cup chopped cabbage)
- Seasoning to taste: salt and pepper

Directions
1. In saucepan, on medium-low heat, cook or steam kidney beans until soft. Drained if needed.
2. In stock pot, in medium-high heat, add cooked beans, carrot, celery, onion, yellow squash, zucchini, cabbage, tomato, and broth. Bring to boil and season with salt, pepper. Reduce to low heat and simmer for 2 hours or up to your flavor consistency.
3. Serve hot with a slice of bread and sprinkle chopped parsley on top. ENJOY!

7. Barley-Chicken Soup

Ingredients
- 4 carrots; removed skin if referred and sliced (about 2 cup)
- 4 celery stalks; chopped (about 2 cup)
- 1 medium onion; peeled and chopped
- 3 quart chicken broth (about 12 cup) [– your choice of broth]
- 2 chicken breasts; skinless, boneless; cut into bite-sized cubes
- 1 tablespoon olive oil (or your choice of fat)
- Seasoning to taste: salt and pepper

Directions
1. In saucepan, on medium-high heat, add ½ tablespoon oil and brown chicken cubes, 3 to 4 minutes. Set it aside.
2. In same saucepan, on medium-high heat, add remaining oil and brown carrots, onion, celery, 5 minutes. Set it aside.
3. In stock pot, on medium-high heat, add chicken, carrot, onion, celery, broth, pearl barley. Bring to boil, season with salt, pepper and stir frequently. Reduce to medium-low heat, simmer with covered, for 1 to 2 hours or until tender and liquid are absorbed. Set aside 5 minutes.
4. Serve hot soup and sprinkle chopped herbs on top if desired.

8. Time-saving Condensed Soup Mix

Ingredients
- 2 cup non-fat milk powder
- ¾ cup cornstarch
- 8 teaspoon (about 8 cubes/ packets) Herb ox Sodium-free Granulated Chicken Bouillon
- 2 tablespoon onion flakes; dried
- 1 teaspoon basil leaves; dried
- 1 teaspoon thyme leaves; dried
- 3 quart water
- Seasoning to taste: salt and pepper

Directions
1. In medium bowl, mix together milk powder, cornstarch, bouillon, onion flakes, basil, and thyme.
2. In stock pot, on medium-high heat, bring water to boil. Add milk-herb-bouillon mix. Cook with stirring constantly until dissolved. Season with salt and pepper if needed.
3. Serve hot/ warm with a slice of bread if desired. ENJOY!
4. Store dried mix in airtight container. Or store as canned soup in fridge.

9. Fresh Veggie Soup

Ingredients
- 2 carrots; cleaned and diced
- 1 celery stalk; diced
- 3 red potatoes; cleaned and cut into quarters
- 1 cup baby spinach;
- 2 small zucchini; cleaned and diced
- 1 cup green beans; rinsed
- 2 tomatoes(or plum/ Italian- your choice); cleaned and chopped
- White part of 1 leek; sliced
- 2 garlic cloves; peeled and minced
- 1 ½ teaspoon thyme leaves; fresh
- 1 teaspoon red pepper flakes
- 9 cup water
- Seasoning to taste: salt and pepper
- 1 tablespoon olive oil

For topping:
- 1 tablespoon olive oil
- 1 cup basil leaves; fresh
- 3 tablespoon parmesan cheese; grated
- Seasoning to taste: salt and pepper

Directions
1. In stock pot, on medium-high heat, brown carrot, potato, leek, celery with oil, garlic, thyme; for 5 to 8 minutes and stir occasionally. Pour water, add zucchini, spinach, green beans, tomatoes and season with salt, pepper, red pepper flakes. Bring to boil and stir frequently, about 5 minutes. Reduce to medium-low heat, cook with covered, for 30 to 45 minutes or until reach your flavor consistency.
2. In food processor, add oil, basil leaves, cheese. Blend to smooth.
3. Serve hot/ warm soup with sprinkle basil-cheese on top if desired. ENJOY!

10. Creamy Chicken-Veggie Soup

Ingredients
- 2 teaspoon oil (your choice of oil)
- 2 chicken breast; skinless and boneless; cut into bite-sized cubes
- 1 ½ cup broccoli; fresh; washed and chopped
- 1 ½ cup cauliflower; fresh; washed and chopped
- 2 carrots; removed skin if referred and chopped
- 1 can (about 10.5 oz) Low-fat cream Broccoli soup
- 1 ¼ cup skim milk
- Seasoning to taste: salt and pepper

Directions
1. In skillet, on medium-high heat, add oil and brown carrot, chicken with oil, season with salt, pepper. Cook with stirring occasionally, for 4 to 5 minutes or until no longer pink with meat.
2. In saucepan, on medium-low heat, pour low-fat broccoli soup, milk and stir to combine. Place chicken, carrot, broccoli, cauliflower and season with salt, pepper. Simmer for 5 to 10 minutes or until vegetables are tender and cooked chicken.
3. Serve hot with a slice of bread or rice if desired. ENJOY!

11. Quick-Served Lentil Soup

Ingredients
- 2 cup lentils; rinsed and drained
- 1 can (about 28 oz.) diced tomatoes
- 3 carrots; removed skin if referred and chopped
- 3 celery stalks; chopped
- 2 cup frozen corn;
- 1 onion; peeled and chopped
- ½ cup soup base (powder) – your choice or use beef soup base as this recipe
- 2 bay leaves
- 2 garlic cloves; peeled and minced
- 6 quarts water
- Seasoning to taste: salt and pepper

Directions
1. In stock pot, on medium-high heat, add lentil, tomato (use whole can), water, bay leaves, and soup base. Bring to boil. Add celery, carrot, onion and season with salt, pepper. Simmer for 10 to 15 minutes or until tender. Be sure to check lentils. Turn off heat, add corn and stir to heat corn a few times. Remove bay leaves.
2. Serve immediately with a cup of brown rice if desired. ENJOY!

12. Quick-Served Chicken Soup

Ingredients
- 2 cans (about 14.5 oz/can) mixed vegetables (or fresh/ frozen- your choice)
- 2 cans (about 10.5 oz/can) cream chicken soup
- 1 package (about 4 medium) medium chicken breast; skinless, boneless; cut into bite-sized cubes
- 2 cup water
- 2 teaspoon oil (optional)

Directions
1. In skillet, on medium-high heat, brown chicken meat with oil, about 3 to 5 minutes or until chicken no longer pink.
2. In stock pot, on high heat, bring water and chicken soup to boil. Reduce to medium heat. Add vegetables, chicken breast and season if needed. Simmer with covered for 15 to 20 minutes or until tender.
3. Serve hot/ warm soup with rice or bread if desired. ENJOY!

13. Quick Chunky Soup

Ingredients
- 1 can (about 15.5 oz) kidney beans; blended if referred
- 3 cans (about 28 oz./can) diced tomatoes
- 2 cans (about 10.5 oz/can) Vegetable Soup
- 2 cup water

Directions
1. In stock pot, on medium-high heat, add tomatoes, vegetable soup, kidney bean and water. Bring to boil. Reduce to medium heat and simmer for 10 to 15 minutes or until reach your flavor consistency.
2. Serve warm soup with sliced of bread or sprinkle grated cheese on top if desired. ENJOY!

14. Turkey-Veggie Pie

Ingredients
- 1 pound ground turkey
- 1 can (about 10.5 oz) Cream chicken soup
- 2 cans (about 14.5 oz/can) mixed vegetables
- 1 tablespoon garlic powder
- 1 package Roasted Garlic Mashed Potatoes
- 1 cup water, hot

Directions
1. Preheat oven to 400 degrees F. grease baking dish with oil.
2. In saucepan, on medium-high heat, brown ground turkey. Drain if needed. Add cream chicken soup, mix vegetables and garlic together to combine. Transfer into baking dish. Set it aside.
3. In food processor, add package mashed potatoes and carefully pour hot water. Mix until combined. Transfer and shape in baking dish on top and cover turkey-veggie perfectly.
4. Bake for 20 minutes or until golden brown on top.
5. Serve hot/ warm with sprinkle herb on top if desired. ENJOY!

15. Turkey-Veggie Soup

Ingredients
- 1 tablespoon oil (your choice of oil)
- 1 onion; peeled and chopped
- 1 celery stalk; chopped
- 2 cup turkey; cooked and chopped
- 4 cup turkey broth (or your choice of broth)
- ½ cup green beans; rinsed and cut into bite-sized long pieces
- ½ cup lima beans; rinsed
- 1 carrot; cleaned and chopped
- ½ cup broccoli; washed and chopped
- ½ cup corn kernels
- 1 small zucchini; cleaned and chopped
- 3 medium tomatoes; cleaned and chopped
- ½ teaspoon dried oregano
- ½ teaspoon dried thyme
- 2 tablespoon parsley leaves; fresh; chopped
- Seasoning to taste: salt and pepper

Directions
1. In a stock pot, on medium-high heat, cook onion, celery with oil until translucent, about 3 minutes. Add turkey, carrot, lima bean, green beans, broccoli, corn kernel, zucchini, tomato, broth, thyme, oregano and season with salt, pepper. Bring to boil, for 8 minutes. Reduce to medium-low heat, simmer for 10 to 12 minutes or until tender veggies.
2. Serve warm soup with rice and sprinkle parsley on top if desired. ENJOY!

16. Thai Inspired Pumpkin Soup

Ingredients
- 1 tablespoon oil (your choice of oil)
- ½ onion; peeled and diced
- 3 celery stalks; chopped
- 3 scallion; peeled and chopped
- 3 cup low-sodium vegetable broth (or your choice)
- 1 can (about 15 oz) solid pumpkin
- 4 tablespoon peanut butter; Thai ginger & red pepper chunky style (or substitute with: peanut butter, minced ginger and red pepper)

Directions
1. In a stock pot, on medium-high heat, brown onion, scallion, celery with oil, about 4 minutes. Add broth, pumpkin. Bring to boil and stir well to incorporate. Blend with hand mixer or transfer into blender until smooth. Add peanut butter and stir well.
2. Serve hot spicy soup with bread and sprinkle paprika powder on top if desired. ENJOY!

17. Oven-Steamed Color Veggies

Ingredients
- 1 yellow squash; cleaned and sliced
- 1 zucchini; washed and sliced
- 2 green/ red pepper (or mix both); removed seed and sliced into strips
- 9 mushrooms; cleaned and sliced
- 1 large onion; peeled and sliced
- ¼ cup oil (your choice of oil)
- 2 tablespoon Lipton soup mix (use Lipton recipe secrets, savory herb with garlic soup mix in this recipe)

Directions
1. Preheat oven to 350 degrees F.
2. In 9 x 13 inch baking pan, toss to cover squash, zucchini, green/ red pepper, mushroom, onion with oil and soup mix. Cover with aluminum foil. Bake for 45 minutes. Take out and mix gently. Bake for more 45 minutes or until tender. Total around 60 to 70 minutes.
3. Serve steamed-oven veggies with mayo and bread if desired. ENJOY!

18. Rich Pumpkin Soup

Ingredients
- 4 potatoes; cleaned, removed skin if referred and chopped
- 1 small carrot; cleaned, removed skin if referred and chopped
- 1 celery stalk; chopped
- ¼ green pepper; removed seed and chopped finely (about 2 tablespoon)
- 2 cup low-sodium chicken broth (or your choice)
- ¼ cup butter; grass-fed
- 2 1/3 cup water
- 1 cup skim milk (or your choice)
- 3 tablespoon flour
- 1 ½ cup pumpkin puree
- 2 teaspoon parsley flakes
- 1 teaspoon sugar
- Seasoning to taste: salt and pepper

Directions
1. In stock pot, on medium-high heat, brown carrot, potato, green pepper, celery about 3 minutes, stir to prevent burned. Add broth, 2 cup water. Bring to boil.
2. Meanwhile, in small bowl, whisk to combine flour with remaining water.
3. Pour flour liquid, pumpkin puree and season with salt, pepper, sugar into soup pot. Stir to incorporate. Reduce to medium-low heat, simmer for 30 minutes or until tender and thicken. Stir milk, parsley into soup and cook for 8 to 10 minutes or until hot.
4. Serve rich soup with slice of bread and sprinkle more parsley on top if desired. ENJOY!

19. Easy Sweet Potato Soup

Ingredients
- 2 sweet potatoes; washed, chopped and soaked into water; drained
- 4 carrots; removed skin if needed and chopped
- 2 sweet pepper; chopped
- 2 leeks; chopped
- 4 celery stalks; chopped
- 2 cubes (about 2 teaspoon) chicken bouillon
- 2 cup water (more or less water is your choice of thickness)
- Seasoning to taste: salt and pepper

Directions
1. In stock pot, on high heat, place sweet potato, carrot, sweet pepper, leeks, celery and pour water until cover veggies. Bring to boil with covered. Reduce to medium-low heat, stir bouillon to incorporate and cook for 40 to 50 minutes or until tender. Blend until smooth or reach your flavor of consistency with hand mixer.
2. Serve hot/ warm sweet potato soup with sprinkle pepper on top if desired. ENJOY!

20. Easy Zucchini Soup

Ingredients
- 2 large zucchini; cleaned and chopped
- 2 large onion; peeled and chopped
- 4 tablespoon oil (your choice)
- 5 cup water
- Seasoning to taste: salt and pepper
- 2 cubes (about 2 teaspoon) chicken bouillon

Directions
1. In stock pot, on medium-high heat, bring water to boil. Stir to incorporate bouillon into water. Add oil, zucchini and onion and season with salt, pepper. Cook about 15 minutes or until tender. Blend with hand mixer to smooth.
2. Serve hot/ warm soup with sprinkle pepper and chopped herb on top if desired. ENJOY!

21. Cheese-Chicken Rice Soup

Ingredients
- 1 can (about 10.5 oz) cream chicken soup
- 1 1/3 cup water
- ¾ cup rice; rinsed
- 1 can (about 14.5 oz) mixed vegetables; drained
- 3 (about 12 oz) medium chicken breasts; boneless, skinless
- 1 cup cheddar cheese; shredded
- ½ teaspoon onion powder
- Seasoning to taste: salt and pepper

Directions
1. Preheat oven to 375 degrees F.
2. In baking dish, mix together water, cream chicken soup, rice, onion and season with salt, pepper. Place chicken breast on top. Cover with aluminum foil and bake for 45 minutes or until cooked.
3. Serve rice and sliced chicken breast, sprinkle cheddar cheese on top if desired. ENJOY!

22. Vegan-Bean Pasta

Ingredients
- 2 tablespoon oil (or your choice of oil)
- 1 small onion; peeled and diced (about ½ cup)
- 1 small zucchini; cleaned and chopped (about ¼ cup)
- ¼ cup frozen green beans
- 1 can (about 15 oz) kidney beans; rinsed, soaked and drained
- 1 can (about 15 oz) small white beans; rinsed, soaked and drained
- 8 oz (about ½ can) diced tomatoes; drained
- 1 small carrot; washed and shredded
- 3 cup baby spinach; fresh
- 4 cup vegetables broth
- 1 ½ cup hot water
- ½ celery stalk; chopped (about ¼ cup)
- 2 garlic cloves; peeled and minced
- 2 tablespoon parsley leaves; chopped
- 1 teaspoon dried oregano
- ½ teaspoon dried basil
- ¼ teaspoon dried thyme
- 1/3 cup shell pasta
- Seasoning to taste: salt and pepper

Directions
1. In saucepan, on medium-high heat, brown onion, celery, green beans, zucchini, garlic with oil, for 5 minutes or until translucent. Add broth, water, tomatoes, white beans, carrot and dried herbs. Bring to boil. Reduce to medium-low heat, simmer with covered for 20 minutes.
2. Uncovered, add spinach leaves, pasta and cook for 20 minutes more or until desired consistency.
3. Serve cooked pasta and vegan sauce with sprinkle cheese or chopped parsley on top if desired. ENJOY!

23. Deer-Corn Pie

Ingredients
- 3 to 5 pound deer meat (use ground meat in this recipe)
- 1 can (family size about 23 oz) mushroom soup
- 2 cans (about 12 oz/can) sweet corn; drained
- 6 cup mashed potato
- 3 cup cheddar cheese (or Copoundy cheese – your choice)

Directions
1. Preheat oven to 375 degrees F.
2. In skillet, on medium-high heat, brown meat for 5 minutes. Transfer into 13 x 9 inch baking dish. Sprinkle corn and pour mushroom soup over deer meat.
3. Meanwhile, in food processor, add package mashed potatoes and carefully pour hot water. Mix until combined. Transfer and shape on baking dish and cover meat-corn. Place shredded cheese on top. Bake for 20 minutes or until golden brown potato. Set it aside to cool, for 5 to 10 minutes.
4. Serve a slice of warm pie with more cheese on top if desired. ENJOY!

24. Mother's Turkey Pasta

Ingredients
- 2 cup turkey meat; diced or shredded – your choice
- 3 cup chicken broth
- 3 cup water
- ½ box (about 8 oz) pasta; cooked and drained
- 1 onion; peeled and chopped
- 4 carrot; frozen; sliced (or fresh- your choice)
- 4 celery stalks; chopped
- 1 teaspoon poultry seasoning (or substitute with dried mix: sage, thyme, marjoram, rosemary, nutmeg and black pepper)
- 1 teaspoon dried oregano
- 1 teaspoon dried basil
- 1 teaspoon garlic powder
- 1 tablespoon parsley flakes
- Seasoning to taste: salt and pepper

Directions
1. In stock pot, on medium-high heat, place turkey, carrot, onion, celery, broth, water and season with salt, pepper, poultry seasoning, oregano, basil, garlic, parsley. Bring to boil. Reduce on medium-low heat, cook with covered for 12 to 15 minutes.
2. Uncover and add cooked pasta. Cook for 5 minutes more or until reach your consistency.
3. Serve pasta and warm/ hot soup with sprinkle grated cheese, chopped fresh herbs if desired. ENJOY!

25. Vegan-Cashew Rice

Ingredients
- 4 carrots; removed skin if needed and chopped
- ½ green cabbage; washed and chopped
- 1 onion; peeled and diced
- 1 apple, removed cored and chopped
- ½ cup cashew; raw; chopped
- ½ cup raisin
- 1/3 cup rice; rinsed and drained
- 2 tablespoon oil (or your choice of oil)
- ¼ cup tomato paste
- 6 cup broth (use vegetable broth in this recipe – your choice)
- Seasoning to taste: salt and pepper

Directions
1. In stock pot, on medium-high heat, add carrot, cabbage, onion and oil. Cook with stirring to prevent burn for 10 minutes.
2. Stir to incorporate broth, tomato paste into pot. Bring to boil. Add and stir apple, rice into veggie-liquid. Reduce to low heat, cook with covered for 30 to 35 minutes.
3. Uncover and stir in cashew, raisin. Cook with covered for 10 minutes more or until rice is tender.
4. Serve rice-veggie with roasted chicken if desired. ENJOY!

26. Cream-Curry Vegan Soup

Ingredients
- 1 teaspoon oil (optional)
- 1 small onion; peeled and diced
- 1 large butternut squash; removed skin, seed and chopped
- 1 large apple; removed core and chopped
- 2 carrots; washed, removed skin if referred and chopped
- 4 cup vegetable broth
- ½ cup almond milk
- 1 bay leaf
- ½ teaspoon nutmeg
- ½ teaspoon curry powder
- Seasoning to taste: salt and pepper

Directions
1. In stock pot, on medium-high heat, brown onion with oil until translucent. Add squash, apple, and carrot and toss to brown with onion, about 4 minutes.
2. Pour broth over vegetables and bring to boil. Reduce to medium-low heat, stir and add bay leaf, nutmeg, curry powder and season with salt, pepper. Simmer with covered for 15 minutes or until soft.
3. Uncover, remove bay leaf. Blend with immersion blender to smooth. Stir to combine almond milk and cook for 10 minutes or until heat through.
4. Serve warm soup with a sliced of bread if desired. ENJOY!

27. Cheesy Vegan Soup

Ingredients
- 1 bay leaf
- 1 serving (about 2 teaspoon) vegetable stock cube
- 1 cup water
- ¾ cup bell pepper; removed seed and sliced
- 1 medium zucchini, washed and sliced
- 2 tomatoes; cleaned and diced
- 3 small potatoes; washed and cut into quarter
- ¾ cup peas; rinsed
- 1 large onion; peeled and chopped
- ¾ cup green beans; washed and cut into bite-sized long pieces
- 1 carrot; cleaned, removed skin if referred and chopped
- 2 cup skim milk
- ½ tablespoon butter; grass-fed
- ½ tablespoon oil (or your choice of oil)
- ½ cup Romano Cheese
- ½ cup Cheddar Cheese
- ¾ teaspoon dried thyme powder
- Seasoning to taste: salt and pepper

Directions
1. In a stock pot, on medium heat, cook onion with butter and oil, about 3 to 4 minutes until translucent. Add potato, carrot, bay leaf, thyme, water, stock cube. Bring to boil. Reduce to medium-low heat, cover and simmer for 5 minutes or until vegetable tender.
2. Uncover, blend until smooth or reach your consistency with immersion blender.
3. Add peas, zucchini, bell pepper, green beans in stock pot. Cook for 5 to 7 minutes or until green beans tender.
4. Pour milk and add cheeses. Stir to incorporate or until heat and smooth soup.
5. Serve hot soup with a slice of bread if desired. ENJOY!

28. Sherry Chicken Soup

Ingredients
- 2 cup chicken; cooked and shredded
- 4 carrots; removed skin and chopped
- 4 celery stalks; chopped
- 1 can (about 14.5 oz) fat-free cream celery soup
- 6 oz skim milk
- 0.5 oz dry sherry wine

Directions
1. In skillet, on high heat, brown celery and carrot, about 4 minutes. Set it aside.
2. In saucepan, on medium-low heat, add chicken, celery, carrot, cream soup, skim milk and wine. Simmer for 10 to 12 minutes or until tender.
3. Serve soup with rice and chopped fresh thyme or parsley on top if desired. ENJOY!

v

Printed in Great Britain
by Amazon